THE POWER OF HOLISTIC HERBAL HEALING

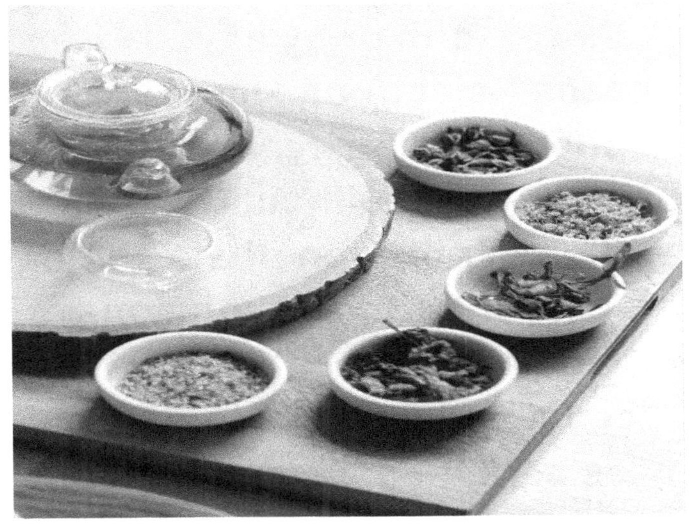

Integrating Nature's Remedies for Wellness

Shamika L. Brad

TABLE OF CONTENT

CHAPTER ONE: INTRODUCTION

The Effectiveness of Natural Curatives

1.0 Knowledge of Herbal Medicine

1.1 Use of traditional herbal remedies throughout history

Traditional usage of herbal remedies indicates extensive historical use, and this is unquestionably true for many items marketed as traditional herbal medicines. A sizable section of the populace in many developing nations depends on traditional healers and their arsenal of medicinal plants to satisfy healthcare demands. Although traditional medicine and contemporary medicine may coexist, herbal remedies often have kept their ubiquity for historical and cultural influences. Commercially speaking, these goods are now more readily accessible, particularly in industrialized nations. In this contemporary environment, substances are sometimes advertised. for purposes never intended by the ancient therapeutic systems from which they were derived. emerged. improves instance, using ephedra (also known as Ma huang) improves athletic performance. Even in certain nations, Herbal medicines are subject to rigorous manufacturing standards. This isn't true everywhere; strict production requirements apply. Germany, where For instance, herbal items marketed as "phytomedicines" are governed by the same standards for quality, safety, and effectiveness as other pharmaceutical goods. In the USA, In contrast, the majority of herbal products are promoted and controlled as nutritional supplements. supplements, a product category where none of these criteria are used to pre-approve items.

1.2 Herbal medicine philosophy

Herbal medicine is comprehensive. The Greek word "holos," which means "whole," is the source of the English term "holistic." It is attending to a person's whole being, including their mind, body, and spirit. Herbal medicine recognizes that every patient is unique and treats the patient, not simply the ailment. By doing this, a customized treatment plan that targets the 'root' of the problem and underlying problems is created for each individual.

1.3 Healing on a Holistic Basis

The holistic approach to healing is a concept and method that acknowledges the interdependence of a person's physical, mental, emotional, and spiritual well-being. The holistic approach looks to understand and treat the full person rather than treating individual health issues. By treating underlying imbalances, supporting the body's intrinsic healing capacities, and encouraging a feeling of empowerment and self-awareness, this complete viewpoint seeks to create balance, harmony, and general well-being.

1.3.1 Fundamental Ideas of the Holistic Healing Method

- The holistic approach recognizes the deep relationship between the mind and body. Physical health may have a big influence on mental and emotional health, and vice versa. The holistic approach seeks to facilitate total healing by addressing psychological elements and emotional emotions.

- Individuality: Everyone has unique physical, emotional, and spiritual characteristics. The holistic approach understands the value of individualized care and adapts treatment programs to the requirements, preferences, and circumstances of each patient.

- The holistic approach seeks to discover and address the underlying causes of health disorders rather than only treating their symptoms. Long-lasting healing might take place by focusing on the underlying reasons rather than the immediate symptoms.

- Wellness and prevention: Holistic healing places a strong emphasis on safeguards for preserving health and well-being. The holistic approach aims to stop sickness in its tracks by encouraging healthy lifestyle choices, stress management, and a balanced diet.

- The holistic approach often incorporates a range of treatment methods, from traditional medicine and herbal medicines to acupuncture, meditation, yoga, and more. This makes it possible to take a multifaceted strategy that meets each person's demands.

- Healing the Whole Person: Holistic healing addresses mental, emotional, and spiritual needs in addition to physical ones. It strives to improve people's quality of life generally and promote change and progress within themselves.

- Empowering people to actively participate in their health journeys is a fundamental tenet of holistic medicine. The ability to make educated choices and actively engage in one's healing process is facilitated by education and self-awareness, which are essential elements.

- Natural treatments and cures that work in harmony with the body's natural cycles and processes are included in many holistic systems. Healing is often supported by the use of mind-body techniques, dietary advice, and herbal therapy.

- Harmony with the Environment: The holistic method often promotes sustainability and environmental awareness. It is thought that positive interaction with the environment enhances general well-being.

- Long-Term healthy: Holistic treatment is more than simply addressing short-term health issues; it also involves promoting a way of life that promotes long-term health. This strategy encourages people to make decisions that will support balance and vitality in the years to come.

The holistic approach makes us aware of the complex network that links every aspect of our existence in a society that often compartmentalizes health and fitness. The holistic treatment provides a route to full well-being by nourishing the physical, mental, emotional, and spiritual aspects of our existence, which is strongly connected with our fundamental need for harmony and balance.

1.4 The Usefulness of Herbal Medicine in the Present Day

The importance of herbal therapy in the current world is still crucial despite a time of tremendous technological growth and modern medical advances. Herbal therapy provides a comprehensive and time-tested strategy that addresses both physical and mental well-being, even though science has changed healthcare.

1.4.1 Here are some reasons why herbal medicine still plays an important role in our contemporary lives

- Herbal therapy relies on millennia of collected knowledge from civilizations all over the globe. **Natural Healing Wisdom**. It provides an understanding of the complex interactions between plants, people, and the environment. This wisdom adds a larger perspective on health and well-being to the understanding of contemporary medicine.

- Herbal medicine has a holistic viewpoint of the person, in contrast to traditional medicine, which focuses on treating symptoms. It acknowledges the interdependence of the physical, mental, and spiritual selves and seeks to correct fundamental imbalances as opposed to only treating symptoms.

- Preventive Care: Prevention is a major focus of herbal medicine. Numerous herbs contain anti-inflammatory properties that assist the body's defensive mechanisms, promoting general health and lowering the risk of chronic disorders.

- Herbal medicine recognizes that each individual is unique, with various constitutions and health requirements. With this individualized approach, herbal treatments may be specifically crafted to address unique situations and promote well-being.

- Compared to pharmaceutical medications, herbal therapies often have fewer negative effects. Many herbs are kinder to the body, lowering the possibility of negative responses and giving individuals looking for natural alternatives an alternative.

- Herbal medicine is firmly ingrained in historical practices and cultural traditions, which is its cultural significance. This link to cultural heritage gives healthcare a significant dimension and encourages a feeling of continuity.

- Herbal therapy may be used in conjunction with conventional therapies as a complementary approach. Numerous medical experts are aware of the possible advantages of using herbal medicines to improve general health and assist the body's natural healing processes.

- Sustainable and Eco-Friendly: As environmental concerns increase, herbal medicine's sustainable and eco-friendly techniques appeal to those looking for all-natural options with the least negative influence on the environment.

- Global Accessibility: People all around the globe often have easier access to herbal cures, particularly in places with less access to modern medical services. Solutions are provided by widely accessible and culturally appropriate local flora and treatments.

- Research and Contemporary Validation: Contemporary research is illuminating the scientific underpinnings of several herbal treatments. The active ingredients and mechanisms of action that support the traditional usage of herbs are being uncovered through studies.

Herbal therapy offers a supplementary route that promotes a stronger relationship with nature and a more holistic perspective of health in a world where synthetic treatments may have unwanted side effects. Herbal medicine should be used with understanding and prudence, but its continued use in the contemporary day is evidence of its persistent ability to improve our general health.

1.5 Recognizing the Interplay of Natural Cure

Understanding the interaction of many components in the natural world that interact intricately to promote healing and well-being is a study into the synergy of nature's medicines. The components of nature's remedies plants, minerals, and other natural substances often have synergistic features that increase their therapeutic benefits, much as ecosystems depend on balance and connectivity. This theory includes the idea that the whole is greater than the sum of its parts and extends beyond the solitary study of individual components.

1.6 Key Considerations in Comprehending the Synergy of Natural Remedies

- The complexity of Natural Substances: Herbs are only one example of a natural remedy that is made up of many different components that all operate together. These substances often interact with one another in ways that strengthen their unique effects, producing a combined therapeutic impact that is greater than what a single substance could accomplish.

- Bioavailability Enhancement: Some substances included in natural medicines may improve other substances' absorption and utilization. This improvement in bioavailability makes sure that the beneficial components are easier for the body to access and use.

- Synergy in natural treatments may have a balanced impact on the body's systems. They can also have modulating effects. For instance, a substance may have a stimulating impact whereas another substance may have a relaxing effect. They combine to provide a well-rounded answer.

- Lower doses of the constituent components may still have the required therapeutic effect because of synergy. This dose decrease may reduce possible negative effects while preserving effectiveness.

- Targeting Multiple Pathways: The natural treatments' synergy often targets different biological pathways. As several facets of health issues are addressed concurrently, this holistic approach may result in a more complete and successful recovery.

- Comparing whole plants to isolated components, whole plants often exhibit synergy since they include a variety of complementary substances. Separating individual substances, however, could not provide the same synergistic results.

- Traditional herbal treatments, often made up of many different plants, have been utilized for millennia owing to their synergistic benefits. These synergies are presently being confirmed by contemporary research scientific investigations.

- Customized mixtures: To optimize synergy, herbalists and practitioners often construct unique mixtures of herbs. These mixtures are customized to meet each person's requirements and health objectives.

- Harmony with Nature: The effectiveness of natural medicines reflects the intrinsic harmony of the surrounding environment. Natural cures survive on the variety and interplay of their constituent parts, much as ecosystems depend on the interaction of many species.

Our awareness of the intricacy and wisdom of the natural world is deepened when we comprehend how the cures found in nature work together. It nudges us to embrace the innate interconnectivity of the components that contribute to our well-being and approach healing with a holistic attitude. Recognizing and honoring the synergistic properties of nature's cures as we work to harness their power may result in more efficient, well-rounded, and long-lasting approaches to health and healing.

PART ONE: Foundations of Herbal Medicine

CHAPTER TWO: Examining Herbal Antibiotics

2.1 Herbal vs. Pharmaceutical Approaches in the Antibacterial Landscape

Herbal and pharmaceutical treatments compete for attention when it comes to treating bacterial illnesses. While both strive to treat bacterial illnesses, they do so via different processes, and comprehending the subtleties of each strategy may provide insightful information about the antibacterial environment.

2.1.1 Herbal methods include:

- Natural Synergy: Herbal treatments often include a complex blend of active ingredients that complement one another. A diverse defense against germs may be developed thanks to this synergy, reducing the likelihood of resistance.

- Broad-Spectrum Action: Rather than focusing on just one kind of bacteria, many herbs have an antibacterial activity that is broad-spectrum in nature. This flexibility is important because different strains of bacteria may cause bacterial illnesses.

- Gentle and Gradual: Compared to pharmaceutical antibiotics, herbal medicines often have a softer effect on the body. As a result, there may be fewer adverse effects and less disturbance of the body's normal microbiome.

- Reduced Resistance Risk: Bacteria may find it more difficult to acquire resistance due to the complexity of herbal medicines. Herbs' diverse chemical composition may prevent germs from developing resistance mechanisms.

- Traditional Knowledge: Traditional medical systems have long used herbal antibacterial treatments. Their effectiveness and importance in the current antibacterial environment are attested to by this historical usage.

- Supporting Immunological Response: Herbal treatments often strengthen the body's immunological response, assisting in the effort to fend against infections in general. Instead of focusing just on germs, this strategy treats the illness as a whole.

2.1.2 Pharmaceutical Techniques:

- Pharmaceutical antibiotics are particularly effective against certain types of bacteria because they are targeted to those strains.

- Pharmaceuticals can provide quick relief, particularly in cases of serious illnesses when quick action is essential.

- Because of the severity or bacterial resistance of certain bacterial illnesses, specialist pharmacological therapies are necessary.

- Widespread Use: Concerns regarding antibiotic resistance have been raised by the excessive and improper use of prescription antibiotics. A threat to world health is the rapid rise of bacterial resistance.

- Pharmaceutical antibiotics have the potential to cause side effects, which may range from minor digestive issues to life-threatening allergic responses.

2.1.3 Complementary methods include:

Many practitioners and researchers support the complementary use of herbal and pharmacological treatments, acknowledging the benefits of both strategies. This strategy combines the herbal remedies' inherent synergy with medicines' focused effects. Herbal medicines may be used to strengthen the body's immune system, lessen the negative effects of prescription antibiotics, and treat bacterial infections holistically.

Both herbal and pharmacological therapies have a place in the ongoing war against bacterial illnesses. Individuals and healthcare professionals may make well-informed choices that support their health objectives by comprehending the advantages and disadvantages of each strategy. This will allow them to consider the possible advantages of natural therapies while also appreciating the advances made in modern medicine.

2.1.4 Finding Your Way Around the World of Herbal Antibiotics

The realm of herbal antibiotics provides a wide and intriguing terrain at an age of rising concern about antibiotic resistance and the demand for natural alternatives. Understanding the fundamentals, choosing, preparing, and using herbal treatments with antibacterial qualities are necessary for navigating this area. This trip illustrates the need of using the healing potential of natural treatments in addition to empowering people to deal with bacterial diseases.

2.1.5 Recognizing the Principles:

- Bioactive chemicals: Plant-based bioactive chemicals are the source of the antibacterial properties of herbal antibiotics. These substances can stop bacterial development, prevent them from reproducing, and even improve the body's immunological response.

- Synergy and Complexity: Many plants contain a mixture of chemicals that combine to operate in synergy to combat germs. This intricacy may prevent germs from becoming resistant.

- Different herbs target different kinds of germs. **Spectrum of Action. Others concentrate on certain strains, while others have broad-spectrum effects. Knowing this range makes it easier to customize treatments for different illnesses.

2.1.6 Choosing the Proper Herbs:

- Before using herbs, it is essential to do a comprehensive study on them. Making educated decisions requires knowledge of the active ingredients, historical use, and compatibility with your medical condition.

- Find out more about herbs including echinacea, oregano, thyme, and garlic that have been shown to have antibacterial effects. Each plant has unique properties that are compatible with certain illnesses.

- Personalization: When choosing herbs, take into account your unique constitution and medical requirements. Depending on the specific qualities of your body, certain herbs may work better for you.

2.1.7 How to Make Herbal Antibiotics

- Herbal antibiotics may be made as tinctures, teas, pills, or topically applied substances. Depending on the qualities of the plant and the preferred manner of administration, each technique has benefits.

- Effectively extracting the herb's active ingredients is a crucial part of good preparation. While teas employ water, tinctures extract via alcohol; each process introduces unique components.

- Follow dose recommendations to guarantee efficacy without running the danger of overuse. Herbalists often provide recommendations for safe and effective usage.

2.1.8 Application and Useful Hints:

- Combining Methods: Herbal antibiotics may be used in conjunction with conventional antibiotics. Combining the two methods in certain circumstances might improve healing and reduce adverse effects.

- Consultation: Seek advice from a licensed herbalist or healthcare professional, particularly if you are managing serious infections or other medical disorders.

- Observation and patience are required since natural therapies may take longer to work than commercially available antibiotics. To get the best outcomes, patience and consistency are crucial.

Learning how to use herbal antibiotics gives you a fascinating chance to incorporate nature's therapeutic knowledge into your health path. You may use herbs' antibacterial power while supporting a holistic approach to health by comprehending the concepts, choosing the right herbs, making efficient preparations, and administering the cures with purpose.

2.1.9 Choosing High-Quality Herbs for Maximum Effect

The quality of the herbs used has a significant impact on the effectiveness of herbal treatments. It's critical to carefully choose herbs that are of the highest quality, are obtained correctly, and are free from impurities to guarantee optimal efficacy and safety. Here is a guide to assist you in choosing high-quality herbs:

1. Source from Credible Vendors:
   - Research Trusted Brands: Seek vendors that have a track record for excellence and openness. Read evaluations and look for suggestions from trustworthy sources.

   - Certifications:Verify the supplier's adherence to Good Manufacturing Practices (GMP) and if their goods are organically grown or otherwise up to par.

   - Ethical Practices: Choose vendors that emphasize fair trading, sustainable harvesting, and ethical sourcing.

2. Evaluation of appearance and senses:

- Visual Inspection: Check the herbs out in person. They should have brilliant colors, be mold-free, and show no contamination-related symptoms.

- Aroma and Taste: Some plants need to have a distinctive scent or taste. Trust your senses; a herb that doesn't have the anticipated flavor or aroma may not be of the highest quality.

3. Plant Identification:

Each plant has a scientific name (Latin name), which guarantees correct identification. Make sure the plant you're looking for is listed under its botanical name.

- Label Transparency: Pick herbs whose labels are clear and contain both botanical and popular names.

Avoid buying anything with unclear or insufficient information.

3. Comparing whole herbs to extracts

- Entire Herbs: By using entire herbs, you may take advantage of the plant's synergistic effects of its many constituents. When making teas or infusions, think about using entire herbs.

- Extracts: Concentrated versions of plants are known as extracts and are often found in tinctures or capsules. Select standardized extracts for their reliable efficacy.

4. Storage and packaging:

- Airtight Containers: Herbs should be stored in airtight containers to prevent deterioration from moisture, air, and light.

- Freshness: Verify the herbs are still fresh and effective by looking at the expiry date.

6. Prevent Contaminants:

- Purity Testing: To be sure that herbs are free of pollutants including pesticides, heavy metals, and microbiological contaminants, choose vendors that carry out independent testing.

- Country of Origin: Use caution if the herbs come from areas with a reputation for having high contamination levels.

7. Consult professionals:

- Herbalists and Practitioners: Consulting with qualified herbalists, naturopaths, or medical professionals may help you choose the best herbs for your needs.

8. Developing Your Own:

- Home Cultivation: If possible, think about cultivating your herbs. You can manage the quality thanks to this from seed to harvest.

An essential step in maximizing the efficacy of herbal treatments is choosing high-quality plants. You may maximize the healing power of nature's friends by picking reliable sources, paying attention to appearance and sensory clues, confirming botanical identification, comprehending the form of herbs, assuring good packing, and avoiding contaminants.

2.2 Making Herbal Antibiotics: Tinctures, Teas, and Other Concoctions

The art of making herbal antibiotics entails choosing the best technique to preserve the effectiveness of the plants while extracting their strong effects. Various approaches each have special benefits that appeal to the tastes and health requirements of the person. Here is a guide on making tinctures, teas, and other kinds of herbal antibiotics:

2.2.1. Tinctures:

Tinctures are potent liquid preparations that effectively bind the medicinal properties of plants. They provide a quick and effective method of taking natural antibiotics.

1. Materials: You'll need premium herbs, brandy or vodka, a glass jar with a tight-fitting cover, labels, and high-quality herbs.

The Process:
- Herbs that have been chopped or powdered should fill the jar, leaving some room at the top.
- The herbs should be fully covered with alcohol.
- For many weeks, shake the jar every day while keeping it in a cold, dark area. Tightly cap the jar.
- After the maceration time, pour the liquid into a clean container using a fine mesh strainer or cheesecloth.
- With the name of the plant, the amount of alcohol, and the date, label the tincture.

2.2.2. Infusions and teas:

Herbal teas and infusions provide a soothing method to take advantage of the antibacterial properties of herbs while also hydrating and soothing the body.

High-quality dried or fresh herbs, boiling water, a teapot or infuser, and a cup are the required ingredients.

The process:
- In a teapot or infuser, pour boiling water over the herbs.
- The suggested steeping period for herbs is normally 5 to 15 minutes.
- Drink the herbal tea after straining the liquid.

2.2.3. Capsules:

When some herbs don't taste good, capsules provide a handy alternative to consuming herbal antibiotics.

High-quality powdered herbs, unfilled vegetarian capsules, and a capsule-filling machine (optional) are required materials.

the process:
- The herb powder should be inserted into the capsule-filling device.
- As directed by the machine, assemble the capsules.
- location the capsules in a cold, dry location after sealing them.

2.2.4. Compresses and poultices:

Poultices and compresses let you administer herbal antibiotics directly to the infected region for external illnesses.

1. Materials: Use hot water, a clean towel, dried or fresh herbs, and bandages (if required).

the process:
- Make a strong decoction or infusion of the plants.
- In the herbal solution, dunk the cloth, and then wring off the extra liquid.
- Apply the cloth to the injured area and, if required, wrap it with a bandage.

2.2.5. Topical Lotions:

Salves provide a method for applying natural antibiotics to the skin while using the advantages of beeswax and carrier oils.

High-quality herbs, carrier oils (such as olive or coconut oil), beeswax, and clean containers are required.

the process:
- Using a gradual heat technique or by leaving the herbs in a sunny location for a few weeks, infuse the herbs in carrier oil.
- After filtering, warm the oil slowly in a double boiler.
- To give the oil a solid consistency, add beeswax.
- After the salve has been poured into clean containers, let it cool and harden.

The technique you select—whether you go with tinctures, teas, capsules, poultices, or salves—depends on your tastes, your medical requirements, and the unique qualities of the herbs you're utilizing. Every technique of preparation provides a different approach to harnessing the antibacterial power of herbs and includes their therapeutic advantages in your regular health practice.

2.3 In-Depth Herb Profiles: A Spotlight on Antibacterial Powerhouses

This sheds light on the incredible antibacterial powerhouses found in nature as we go further into the field of herbal medicines. You'll obtain a thorough grasp of the therapeutic potential and uses of certain herbs by investigating their unique traits and characteristics. Each herb description provides details on its historical use, active ingredients, preparation techniques, and useful advice for the best outcomes.

2.3.1 Allium sativum, or garlic, is a natural protector of health.

- **Historical Use:** Learn why garlic has been prized for generations as a powerful antibacterial agent that may treat a variety of ailments.

- **Active Compounds:** Discover the essential substances, including allicin, that give garlic its strong antibacterial and immune-boosting effects.

Learn how to make garlic into a tincture, tea, or topical treatment, and discover the advantages of raw vs cooked garlic.

- **Practical Tips:** Find unique methods to use garlic in your diet and everyday activities to maximize its antimicrobial effects.

2.3.2 Immune-Boosting Warrior: Echinacea (Echinacea spp).

Explore the Native American customs that acknowledged echinacea's function in enhancing the immune system and preventing illnesses.

- Active Compounds: Learn about the polysaccharides and alkamides in echinacea and how they affect the immune system.

- Preparation Methods:Learn to use echinacea to make tinctures, teas, and infusions to benefit your immune system.

- Practical Tips: Discover when and how to use echinacea to strengthen general immunity and help your body's defenses against bacterial illnesses.

2.3.3 Hydrastis canadensis, sometimes known as goldenseal

- Historical Use: Learn how Native Americans used goldenseal for its significant antibacterial and anti-inflammatory effects.

Discover the alkaloids, such as berberine, that give goldenseal its potent antibacterial properties under the section titled "Active Compounds."

- Preparation Methods: Discover how to make topical treatments and tinctures from goldenseal to fight infections and encourage recovery.

- Practical Tips: Learn about the function of goldenseal in treating respiratory, intestinal, and skin illnesses while taking sustainability into account.

2.3.4. Thyme (Thymus vulgaris): A Healing Herb in the Kitchen

- Historical Use: Travel back in time to see how thyme was used as an antiseptic and treatment for respiratory problems.

Explore the volatile oils found in thyme, such as thymol, to learn more about its significant antibacterial and antiseptic properties.

- Preparation Methods: Learn to make thyme-infused teas, oils, and steam inhalations to help with respiratory health and treat infections.

- Practical Tips: Make the most of thyme's culinary diversity by including it in your diet and using it topically to treat a variety of illnesses.

You'll acquire a whole toolset of antibacterial superpowers that can be used to fight infections, improve immunity, and advance holistic well-being by exploring these in-depth herb profiles. You'll be prepared to make wise choices about including these herbal medicines in your quest for better health as you investigate the distinctive qualities and uses of each plant.

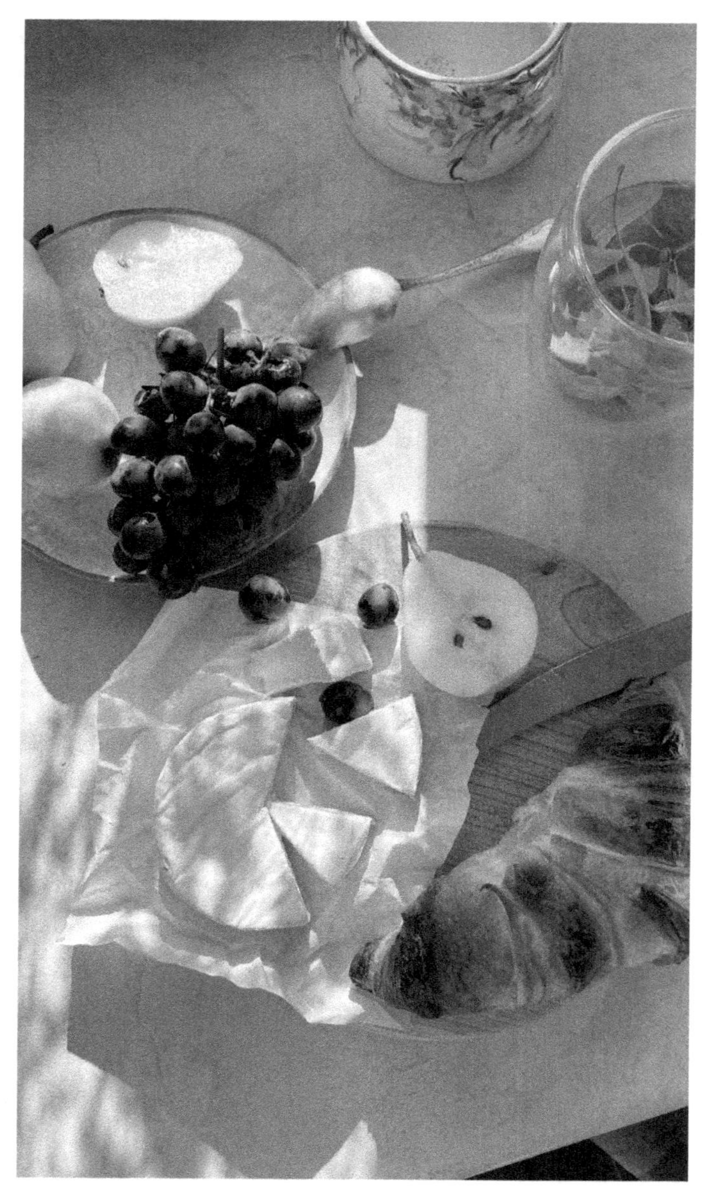

CHAPTER THREE: Navigating the Modern Herbal Dispensary

3.1 Identifying herbs and ethical harvesting

The contemporary herbal pharmacy has a strong connection with the plant world at its core. To build a stronger connection with nature and ensure the sustainability of herbal resources, this chapter digs into the critical abilities of herbal identification and ethical harvesting. By understanding these fundamental techniques, you'll start a journey beyond treatments and be able to work with plants as partners in your quest for well-being.

3.1.1 The Science of Herbal Detection:

- Botanical Exploration: Start by developing your capacity to distinguish between various plant species based on their leaves, blooms, stems, and other distinguishing characteristics.

- Botanical Field Guides: Learn about the importance of botanical field guides and other resources that provide in-depth descriptions, illustrations, and photos for precise identification.

- Local Ecosystems: Recognize the significance of comprehending your local ecosystems, since plants often flourish in particular settings, which contributes to their distinctive characteristics.

3.1.2. Sustainable agriculture and ethical harvesting:

- Respectful Harvesting: Acquire knowledge of the ethical harvesting principles, stressing the significance of taking just what is required and maintaining the integrity of the environment.

- Cultivation and Conservation: Learn about the advantages of growing your herbs at home to promote local biodiversity and help protect wild plant populations.

- Harvesting Seasons: Appreciate the value of gathering plants at their peak times to preserve their health and potency for therapeutic usage.

3.1.3. Deepening Your Relationship with Plants:

- Mindful Observation: Master the skill of mindful observation by using all of your senses to connect deeply with plants and develop an understanding of their healing potential.

- Ceremony and Gratitude: Adopt the custom of participating in rituals or ceremonies that honor plants and show appreciation for their offerings.

- Cultivating Relationships: Develop a reciprocal connection with plants by nurturing a dynamic relationship that goes beyond utilitarianism and recognizes the wisdom they have to share.

3.1.4. Considering Your Stewardship:

- Wildcrafting Ethics: Recognize the ethics of wildcrafting and strike a balance between the need to protect natural habitats and the demand for herbal resources.

- Conservation Efforts: Examine the function of conservation groups and programs devoted to safeguarding and maintaining indigenous plant species.

- Sharing Knowledge: Give back to society by imparting your understanding of herbal classification, moral harvesting, and environmentally friendly methods.

You'll start a voyage of intimate connection with plant life in this chapter. You may develop the ability to properly obtain medicinal resources while simultaneously developing close contact with nature if you become an expert at herbal identification, adopt ethical harvesting methods, and nurture a deeper connection with plants. Keep in mind that your trip into the plant kingdom goes beyond finding treatments; it's a lifetime connection that enhances your well-being and contributes to the peace on our planet as you traverse the contemporary herbal pharmacy.

3.2 Extracts, infusions, decoctions, and other herbal preparations are made.

Disclosing the Science of Herbal Extraction In the field of herbal medicine, artistry is the skillful extraction of plant essence to produce strong treatments. The procedures used to turn unprocessed plant material into potent therapeutic solutions are revealed in this chapter's section on herbal extraction. You'll be able to produce treatments that capture the vivacity and brightness of nature's abundance after you master these approaches.

3.2.1. The Vitality of Extraction:

- Extraction Methods: Learn about the many processes used to draw out the medicinal properties of plants, such as maceration, percolation, and expression.

- Solvents: Investigate the function that solvents, such as water and alcohol, play in releasing the active components of plant material.

- Selecting the Right technique: Recognize how the plant, its characteristics, and the intended result influence the extraction technique of choice.

3.2.2. How To make herbal tinctures:

Learn the step-by-step procedure for making alcohol-based tinctures, in which alcohol serves as a powerful solvent to extract the chemicals from the plant.

- Extracting Active Constituents: Learn how alcohol efficiently extracts both oil- and water-soluble substances to produce a concentrated herbal medicine.

- Alcohol Percentage: Recognize the significance of selecting the appropriate alcohol percentage for various herbs and their intended effects.

3.2.3. Making Herbal Infusions and Teas:

- Water-Based Extraction: Discover the world of herbal teas and infusions, where a variety of plant chemicals are extracted using hot water.

- Differentiate between teas and infusions, with teas requiring shorter steeping durations and infusions requiring longer steeping times to extract more sensitive ingredients.

- Creating Balanced Blends: Discover the technique of mixing herbs to produce delicious infusions and teas that have medicinal properties.

3.2.4. How to Prepare Herbal Decoctions

- Concentrated Brews: Gain knowledge of the creation of decoctions, which are made by simmering herbs in water to draw out their harder, more robust components.

- Ideal for Roots and Barks: Learn that decoctions are very useful for drawing out chemicals from plant roots and barks.

- Improving Extraction: Investigate methods to improve extraction, such as longer simmering and covering the pot to stop evaporation.

3.2.5. Beyond Solvents Extracts:

- Oil-Based Infusions: Learn about herbal-infused oils, which are made by steeping herbs in carrier oils to extract their medicinal characteristics for topical use.

Learn about alternate extraction techniques including making glycerites (using glycerin) and herbal vinegar (using vinegar), each of which has its advantages and uses.

3.2.6. Combining science with the arts:

- customization: Recognize how the technique of making herbal extracts allows for customization as you create treatments that are tailored to your unique medical requirements.

- Experimentation: To find your preferred treatments, embrace the creative part of herbal extraction by trying various procedures and ratios.

3.2.7. Preservation and Storage:

- Maintaining Potency: Discover the best storage practices to use to guarantee that your herbal extracts retain their potency and effectiveness throughout time.

Examine the significance of utilizing opaque dark glass containers to shield your extracts from light and preserve their quality.

Through this investigation of the craft of herbal extraction, you'll learn how to make powerful medications that capture the essence of plants. Each technique provides a different means of capturing nature's therapeutic potential, whether it be via the creation of tinctures, teas, decoctions, or oil infusions. By learning these methods, you'll be able to harness plant energy for your overall well-being and become a custodian of old herbal knowledge.

3.3 Finding the Right Balance: Unlocking the Art of Dosage

Dosing is an art in herbal therapy that calls for accuracy, intuition, and knowledge of each patient's requirements. This chapter's part goes deeply into the subtleties of herbal doses, assisting you in achieving the fine line between maximizing medicinal benefits and guaranteeing safety. You'll be able to navigate the complex world of herbal treatments with assurance and awareness if you learn the art of dose.

3.3.1. Dosing: A Customized Approach:

- Individual Variability: Learn how characteristics like age, weight, health, and sensitivity affect how much medication is needed for each person.

- Starting Low and Slow: Recognize the idea of beginning with a low dosage and gradually increasing it to see how your body reacts to the herbal medicine.

- Seeking Professional Guidance: Appreciate the importance of speaking with a licensed herbalist or healthcare professional to get individualized dose advice.

3.3.2. Herbal Dosage Forms: Investigating Your Options

- Tinctures: Gain knowledge on how to determine the dose when using tinctures, taking into account the herb's strength and the amount of alcohol present.

- Teas and Infusions: Learn how to calculate dose while making herbal teas and infusions, taking the herb's potency and intended medicinal impact into account.

- Capsules and Tablets: Consider the dosage for herbal capsules and tablets to make sure the concentration of the active

ingredients is in line with your health
objectives.

3.3.3. Administration: Timing Is Important:

- Frequent Small Doses: Acquaint yourself with the idea of frequent dosing with smaller doses, especially for acute diseases, to sustain an active compound's constant presence.

- Spaced Dosing: Recognize the benefits of spaced dosing, which calls for higher dosages to be given less often and is typically appropriate for chronic diseases.

- Timing with Meals: Learn how the effectiveness and absorption of herbal treatments might be affected by taking them before or after meals.

3.3.4. Adapting to Various Stages:

- Initial Phase: Consider using greater initial dosages during an illness's acute phase, then gradually reducing them as symptoms subside.

- Maintenance Phase: Recognize the change to a lower maintenance dosage to maintain improvements and avoid overuse.

3.3.5. Observing and modifying:

- Listening to Your Body: Adopt the discipline of paying attention to how your body reacts to the herbal cure and modify it as necessary.

- Keeping a diary: Think about keeping a dosing diary to record your experiences and aid in dosage adjustment over time.

3.3.6. Special Populations to Be Considered:

- Children and Elderly: Find out about dosing concerns for these groups of people, since their physiology may call for different amounts.

- Pregnancy and Lactation: Recognize the warnings and guidelines for using herbs when pregnant or nursing.

3.3.7. Developing Patience: Juggling Rapid Progress and Gradual Recovery:

- Immediate vs. Gradual: Recognize the delicate balance between wanting outcomes right now and giving herbs time to develop gradually, supporting the body's natural healing processes.

- Regular Consistency: Recognize the value of regular dosage over time, even if no improvements are seen right away.

You'll traverse the world of herbal medicines with competence and awareness after you've mastered the art of dose. You may empower yourself to fully use the benefits of natural treatments while preserving your health by finding the perfect balance for each person, taking dosage forms, frequency, and time into consideration, and adjusting to various phases. Dosage is a harmonic interplay between you and the healing power of plants; it is not just a number figure, keep that in mind.

3.4 Ensuring Safety: Herb-Drug Interactions and Contraindications

Safety is of utmost importance in the field of herbal medicine. Understanding possible contraindications and herb-drug interactions is the main topic of this chapter's part, which helps you embark on a safe and risk-free herbal journey. By negotiating these complexities, you'll equip yourself to make wise decisions that put your health first and seamlessly combine herbal medicines with other medical procedures.

3.4.1. Exceptions: When Herbs Should Not Be Used:

- Individual Health problems: To ensure that you steer clear of any possible issues, educate yourself on any particular medical problems or circumstances that would make using a certain plant contraindicated.

- Pregnancy and Lactation: Recognize the herbs that are not advised owing to their possible effects on maternal and fetal health during pregnancy and lactation.

- Allergies and Sensitivities: Learn how using particular herbs may need to be avoided if you have allergies or sensitivities to them, to avoid negative effects.

3.4.2. Navigating Complexity in Herb-Drug Interactions:

- Complex Interaction Mechanisms: Recognize the different ways in which herbs and prescription medications may interact, influencing absorption, metabolism, and effectiveness.

- Contact with Healthcare Providers: Recognize the value of open contact with healthcare professionals to address any possible herb-drug interactions, particularly if you're taking medication.

- Influences on Absorption and Metabolism: Examine how herbs may affect a drug's absorption and metabolism, affecting how effective it is or maybe even having unfavorable consequences.

3.4.3. Reliable Resources for Researching Interactions Include:

- Herb-Drug Interaction Databases: Find reliable websites and databases that provide details on possible interactions between herbal remedies and prescription medications.

- Herbalists and Healthcare Professionals: Consult with qualified herbalists and healthcare professionals who are familiar with herb-drug interactions for advice.

3.4.4. Timing and Distancing: Reducing Interactions:

- Spacing doses: Discover the practice of separating the dosages of herbs and pharmaceuticals to reduce the possibility of interactions and guarantee adequate absorption.

- Discussing Options: Speak with medical professionals about changing prescription doses or looking into other herbs to reduce interactions.

3.4.5. An ongoing process of monitoring and vigilance

- Observing Your Body: Adopt the habit of paying great attention to your body's reactions whenever you combine new herbs with prescription meds.

- frequent Check-Ins: Arrange frequent check-ins with your doctor to see how herbal treatments are affecting your health and to make any required modifications.

3.4.6. A Holistic Approach: Weighing Risks and Benefits:

- Educated Decision-Making: Be aware that including herbs in your health regimen necessitates making educated choices that weigh possible advantages against potential hazards.

- Individualized Approach: Recognize the individuality of your body and health circumstances and personalize your herbal selections to meet your requirements.

A critical part of your trip is learning how to travel across the herbal medicine landscape of safety. You'll build a foundation of knowledge that enables you to successfully include herbs into your health routines by comprehending contraindications, respecting the intricacy of herb-drug interactions, finding out trustworthy resources, and adopting a holistic approach. Remember that safety is a continuous process, and your dedication to comprehending and minimizing possible hazards will guarantee a successful and pleasant herbal trip.

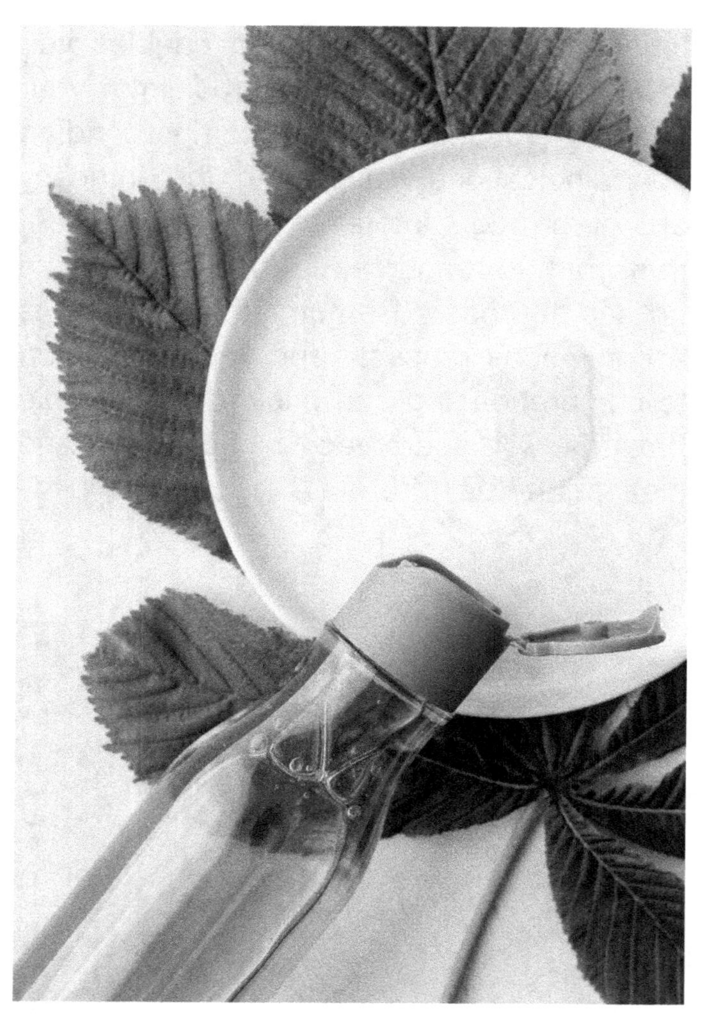

PART TWO

ENCYCLOPEDIA OF HERBS

CHAPTER FOUR: Encyclopedia of Herbal Remedies

4.1 Dive into 550 herbs: Botanical Description and Characteristics

In this long chapter, we begin our journey through the rich tapestry of the plant kingdom. Focusing on 550 herbs, each with unique qualities and potential healing properties, this section serves as a definitive guide to the world of herbal remedies. Through the descriptions, characteristics, and history of plant use, you will gain a deeper understanding of the different herbs that nature has bestowed upon us.

4.1.1. Botanical Description:

Latin name: Dive into the botanical world by discovering the Latin name for each herb, providing a standardized way to identify and communicate about them.

- Family and Gender:Explore the family and genus of each herb, providing insight into their botanical relationships.

- Common name: Learn the common names by which these herbs are known in cultures, regions, and traditions.

4.1.2. Forms and habits:

- Factory structure: Explore the morphology of each herb, including details of leaves, stems, flowers, and fruits, painting a vivid picture of their physical characteristics.

- Growth habits: Understand grass as annuals, perennials, shrubs, or trees, providing detailed information about the grass's lifespan and growth pattern.

4.1.3. Indigenous regions and habitats:

- Geographic origin: Explore the regions of origin of each herb, highlighting the environment in which they grow.

- Habitat options: Explore the habitats where these herbs grow naturally, from lush forests to arid deserts.

4.1.4. Using history and folklore:

- Ancestral wisdom: Explore the history of each herb's use in different systems of traditional medicine, providing insight into their proven healing applications.

- Cultural significance: Explore the folklore and cultural significance attached to these herbs, revealing their role in rituals, ceremonies, and storytelling.

4.1.5. Therapeutic properties:

- Medical benefits: Dive into the specific therapeutic properties of each herb, such as anti-inflammatory, analgesic, diuretic, and more.

- Potential use: Understand the diseases and conditions for which each herb has been traditionally used, giving an overview of their potential applications.

4.1.6. Preparation and dosage:

- Form and Dosage: Learn about the different forms each herb can be prepared in, from teas and tinctures to poultices and ointments.

- Dosage Instructions: Know the recommended dosage for each herb, guiding you through the art of creating safe and effective remedies.

4.1.7. Precautions and Contraindications:

- Security Considerations: Discover the potential precautions and contraindications associated with each herb, allowing you to make an informed decision.

- Interact: Understand all known herbal and pharmaceutical drug interactions to ensure your well-being.

4.1.8. Cultivation and Harvest:

- Cultivation tips: Learn how to grow each herb in your garden, fostering a deeper connection with nature and sustainable practices.

- Harvest period: Understand the optimal time to harvest different parts of the grass, ensuring maximum capacity.

As you embark on this comprehensive journey through 550 herbs, you'll have an invaluable resource to use as your herbal encyclopedia. Each entry encapsulates the essence of the plant's identity, potential healing properties, and its place in the world. This section opens the door to a treasure trove of natural remedies, inviting you to explore, learn and incorporate the wisdom of the plant kingdom into your wellness journey.

4.2 Examining Folklore and Traditional Uses

In this section, we set off on an intriguing trip through the rich tapestry of folklore and traditional applications connected to the amazing world of herbal treatments. We unearth a wealth of old knowledge that has been handed down through the ages as we investigate the cultural and historical value of several plants.

4.2.1 Understanding ancient knowledge

Herbal treatments have played a significant role in human history and have been profoundly ingrained in many different cultures and civilizations. We'll dig into the ancient wisdom that helped our forefathers comprehend the curative powers of plants. We'll learn how civilizations throughout the world have used plants to treat illnesses, from Native American cures to Ayurvedic practices.

4.2.2 Folklore and Healing Stories

Herbs have long been associated with myths, folklore, and stories that illustrate the close relationship between people and the environment. We'll get completely engrossed in the legends that have shaped herbal folklore, from the ethereal qualities of rare herbs to the superstitions related to certain plants. These tales provide insights into prehistoric beliefs in addition to illuminating the fundamental worth of herbal treatments in diverse communities.

4.2.3 Using herbs in ceremonies and rituals

As conduits between the earthly and the divine, many plants have been essential in holy rites and ceremonies. We'll look at how plants were employed in rituals for healing, safety, and spiritual ties. We'll reveal the spiritual qualities that have influenced herbal traditions throughout time, whether smudging with sage or adding herbs to ceremonial beverages.

4.2.4 Cultural Customs and Traditions

Every culture approaches herbal medicine differently, influenced by its environment, beliefs, and resources. We'll explore several techniques that have impacted the development of herbalism, from the intricate plant mixtures used in Chinese Traditional Medicine to European herbal traditions. We'll discuss important plants from different civilizations and how their holistic advantages have led to their veneration.

4.2.5 The Knowledge of Ancient Recipes

History is replete with handwritten cures and recipes developed by previous generations. We'll unearth these venerable concoctions that have been handed down through generations, revealing the synergistic combinations that were used to treat typical maladies. We'll also look at how well historical recipes fit into contemporary environments.

We will develop a greater respect for the cultural legacy that shapes our knowledge of herbal treatments via this investigation of traditional applications and folklore. Join us as we explore the ties that bind us to the wisdom of our ancestors and celebrate the timeless lessons that still hold in today's society.

4.3 Active Substances and Mechanisms in the Science of Herbal Healing

We set out on a tour through the complex realm of the science underpinning herbal medicine in this chapter. We'll look into the ways by which these chemicals interact with the human body to promote well-being as well as the active ingredients that give herbs their unique medicinal capabilities.

4.3.1 The Nature's Pharmacy Unveiling:

Herbs are more than simply haphazard plants; they are complex reservoirs of bioactive substances that have enormous effects on our bodies. We'll explore the many kinds of substances present in herbs, including phenolic compounds, alkaloids, flavonoids, and terpenoids. We'll look at how certain substances, such as the anthocyanins in blueberries and the polyphenols in green tea, contribute to the rich variety of herbal treatments.

4.3.2 The Pharmacokinetic Dance:

Understanding the body's absorption, metabolization, and elimination of herbal substances is essential to understanding their effects. We'll explore terms like bioavailability, distribution, metabolism, and excretion as we dig into the field of pharmacokinetics. This information sheds light on how herbs move through our systems to have a medicinal effect.

4.3.3 Molecular Signaling and Receptor Binding in Cellular Communication

Herbal substances interact intricately with receptors and signaling cascades at the cellular level. We'll explore the complex interactions between herbal substances and enzymes, cell surface receptors, and receptors for neurotransmitters. We'll look at how herbs may alter cellular communication and affect physiological reactions, from agonists to antagonists.

4.3.4 Targeting Oxidative Stress and Inflammation

Oxidative stress and inflammation are major contributors to a wide range of health issues. We'll look at the ways through which herbal components reduce cellular damage and promote general health, as well as how they have anti-inflammatory and antioxidant qualities. We'll explore nature's armory of anti-inflammatory substances, from the curcumin in turmeric to the resveratrol in grapes.

- Adapting to Stress: Adaptogens' Function:

Herbs that help the body adapt to stress and preserve equilibrium are known as adaptogenic herbs, and they occupy a special position in herbal therapy. We'll look at how these herbs affect the sympathetic nervous system and the hypothalamic-pituitary-adrenal axis to boost resilience in the face of stress. We'll comprehend how adaptogens support homeostasis using examples like ashwagandha and holy basil.

- Herbal Synergy Unlocked: The Entourage Effect

Herbs often show greater therapeutic benefits when their diverse constituents combine synergistically, much as an orchestra's instruments make harmonious music when they perform together. We'll go into the idea of the entourage effect to see how the interactions between various components in a plant might boost its therapeutic potential.

- Research and Clinical Evidence: Validation via Tradition and Modernization

Traditional herbal usage is being supported by thorough study as science develops. We'll look at research that explains how herbal remedies work, from how they affect gene expression to how they affect cellular pathways. We'll talk about the value of evidence-based herbal therapy and how research is advancing our knowledge.

Investigating the science underlying herbal remedies helps us better understand the complex web of interactions that herbs have with our bodies. Join us as we bridge the gap between conventional thinking and cutting-edge scientific understanding as we discover the secrets of herbal substances and processes.

4.4 Real-World Applications: Each Herb's Health Benefits

With the information and direction to use each herb's therapeutic potential for your well-being, we go from the world of theory to practical practice in this chapter. You'll learn how to use these botanical jewels in your everyday life to manage a range of health issues as we go through this section.

4.4.1 Making herbal teas and infusions:

Discover the technique of making herbal teas and infusions, a time-honored practice that enables you to consume the benefits of herbs in liquid form. Learn the fine art of appropriate brewing, dosage, and preparation methods to extract the full range of beneficial components. We'll walk you through the procedure whether you want chamomile for relaxation or nettle for nutrient absorption.

- Tinctures: Concentrated Natural Elixirs: Learn about tinctures, strong liquid extracts that distill the essence of botanicals in glycerin or alcohol. Explore the techniques for creating tinctures at home and learn the best plant extraction ratios. Discover how to use the concentrated power of herbal tinctures, from valerian for sleep to echinacea for immune support.

- Topical applications, balms, and salves: In addition to providing internal assistance, herbs are essential companions for maintaining exterior well-being. Investigate the world of skin-care products made from herbal salves, lotions, and balms. We'll walk you through making herbal remedies for topical use, using calendula to soothe irritated skin and arnica to ease aching muscles.

- Cooking Magic: Including Herbs in Common Dishes: Herbs may enhance your culinary creativity and are not only for the medicinal cupboard. Learn how to use herbs in typical foods to enhance taste and offer nutritional value. We'll examine the art of culinary herbalism to improve both flavor and well-being, whether it is using thyme in soups or rosemary in roasted veggies.

- Herbs Integrated Into Lifestyle Rituals: You may include herbs in your everyday rituals and activities. Learn how to include herbs into your lifestyle, whether it be by drinking herbal tea to start your day, utilizing aromatherapy to set the tone, or using herbs to support mindfulness practices. We'll show you how to integrate herbs into your holistic way of living.

- Personalized Herbal Blends: Meeting Your Individual Needs: Every person's path to health is different. Discover how to make custom herbal concoctions that are suited to your requirements. Whether your health objectives are digestive balance, immunological support, or stress reduction, we'll provide advice on how to choose and combine herbs to create blends that are in line with your needs.

- Connecting with Nature Through Harvesting and Foraging: We'll look at the skill of ethically gathering and foraging for herbs for individuals who have a stronger connection with the natural world. Learn the principles and methods of wildcrafting and how to recognize, collect, and prepare wild herbs for personal use. We'll promote a broader understanding of the relationship between people and plant life.

You'll develop the abilities and confidence to start your herbal practice as we dive into practical applications. You may empower yourself to develop well-being, treat health issues, and create a peaceful connection with the therapeutic gifts that nature offers by adopting the practical knowledge of herbalism. Come along with us as we set out on this practical road to comprehensive well-being.

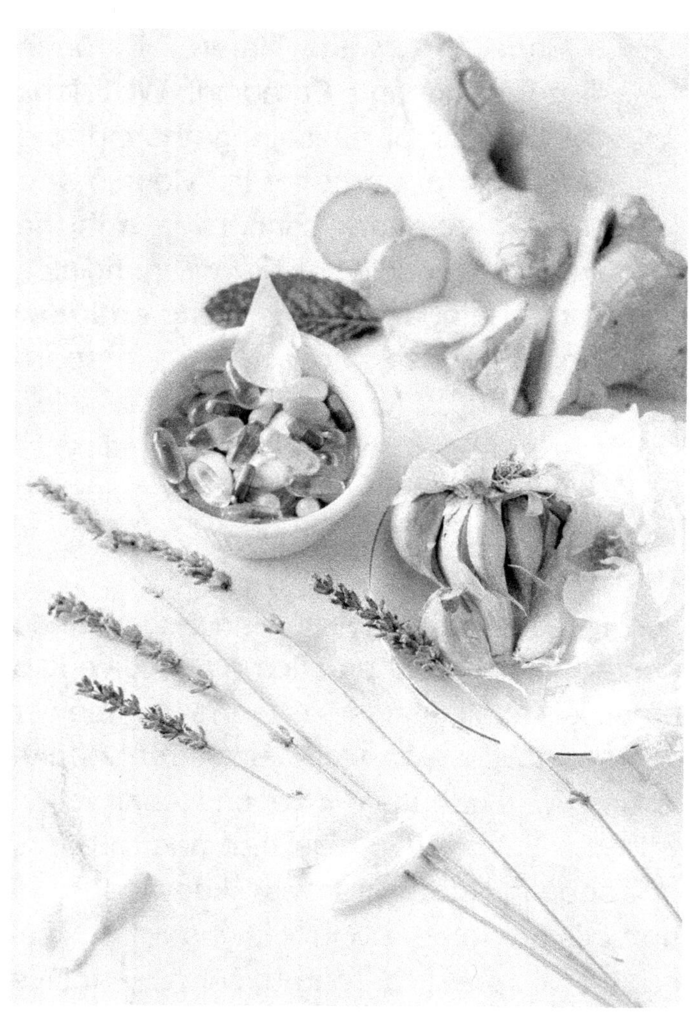

CHAPTER FIVE: Herbal First Aid: Nature's Healing Touch

5.1 Using Herbal Care to Treat Cuts, Burns, and Bruises

In this chapter, we explore the world of herbal first aid, where nature's curative powers provide comfort and treatment for common wounds and illnesses. We will provide you with the knowledge to react to wounds, burns, and bruises with the healing power of nature as we examine the mild but potent treatments that herbs offer.

A holistic approach to comprehending herbal first aid is as follows:
Herbs may be your partners in delivering instant comfort and assisting the body's natural healing processes when accidents occur. We'll give you an introduction to the holistic ideas that underpin herbal first aid, emphasizing not just physical recovery but also mental well-being in trying times.

Herbal antiseptics and healing agents for cuts and wounds
Find herbal heroes that can clean cuts and wounds and hasten their recovery. We'll lead you in choosing herbs that help with infection prevention and tissue regeneration, from calendula's calming benefits to lavender's antibacterial powers.

5.1.1 Cooling and Calming Herbs for Burn Healing

Herbs provide a soothing balm for sensitive skin despite the discomfort and anguish that burns may cause. Learn about the plants that may soothe burns, from the cooling gel of aloe vera to the healing qualities of comfrey. Learn how to make herbal remedies that reduce pain and aid in recovery.

5.1.2 Herbal Recovery and Comfort for Bruises and Contusions

Although bruises and contusions may be unattractive and inconvenient, herbs can help them heal more quickly. Learn about herbs like arnica and witch hazel that promote healthy circulation and relieve inflammation. We'll help you create topical treatments that help with edema and discoloration reduction.

5.1.3 Making a Herbal First Aid Kit: Supplies Every Home Should Have

Create a herbal first aid kit that is stocked with adaptable treatments to be ready for unforeseen circumstances. We'll help you put up a selection of tinctures, oils, salves, and tinctures that can treat a range of wounds and illnesses. Your kit will grow to be a dependable ally in difficult times.

5.1.4 Increasing Self-Assurance in Herbal Response: Useful Applications

We'll provide you with the knowledge and skills necessary to successfully use herbal medicines to treat wounds, burns, and bruises via practical advice and detailed instructions. We'll provide you with the knowledge and skills you need to give compassionate and efficient treatment, whether it's making a poultice for a small wound or using a herbal salve on a burn.

5.1.5 The Whole Family Can Benefit from Herbal First Aid

Herbs are not only mild enough for every member of your family, but they are also safe. We'll go through how to use herbal first-aid medicines for kids, adults, and even pets so that your loved ones may benefit from nature's healing power when they're in need.

Join us as we go to the center of herbal first aid, where the demands of common injuries are met by the knowledge of plant life. Through this investigation, you'll develop the capacity to provide solace, relief, and healing to yourself and your loved ones, reinforcing the strong connection between people and nature's therapeutic gifts.

5.2 Rapid Pain Management and Inflammation Control

We go more deeply into the field of herbal first aid in this chapter, concentrating on quick pain alleviation and successful inflammation treatment. You'll learn how to naturally treat pain and decrease inflammation by using the power of herbs.

5.2.1 Herbal Insights: Understanding Pain and Inflammation

Herbs may provide a comprehensive approach to controlling both pain and inflammation, which often go hand in hand. Examining how herbal components may influence these processes without the negative effects sometimes associated with conventional drugs, we'll dig into the basic causes of pain and inflammation.

5.2.2 Nature's Analgesics: Herbs for Pain Relief

Learn about the natural painkillers that may help with different kinds of pain. We'll introduce you to herbs that may aid with pain relief, whether it's from headaches, muscular pains, or minor injuries, from salicin in willow bark to the calming properties of Jamaican dogwood.

5.2.3 Herbs that reduce inflammation naturally include

The body responds to harm with inflammation, but when it persists for a long time, it may cause some health problems. Learn about the plants that have anti-inflammatory characteristics to control the body's inflammatory reaction. We'll examine plants with various therapeutic properties, such as turmeric, ginger, and boswellia.

5.2.4 Making Balms, Liniments, and Oils for Herbal Pain Relievers

Learn how to prepare herbal preparations for topical use that reduce localized discomfort. We'll help you choose the best herbs and develop formulas that provide precise relief whether you're making a herbal balm, liniment, or infused oil. For quick treatment, these formulations may be immediately administered to sore spots.

5.2.5 Teas and Decoctions: The Art of Herbal Infusions for Pain and Inflammation

Explore the world of herbal infusions, which may treat internal discomfort and inflammation. We'll show you how to make herbal teas and concoctions that you can enjoy all day long. We'll look at herbs that promote general wellness, such as chamomile for calming the nerves and willow bark for pain treatment.

5.2.6 Finding the Right Balance for Considerations Regarding Dosage and Safety:

Knowing the right dose for herbal medicines is essential for pain relief that works without side effects. We'll go through how to calculate the ideal dose for various herbs and how to keep an eye on your body's reaction. We will also look at security issues and possible interactions.

5.2.7 Self-Care Empowerment: Making Knowledgeable Decisions

You will acquire the information and skills necessary to make wise decisions about your health as you delve further into the field of herbal first aid for pain and inflammation. You'll promote a feeling of strength and inborn resilience by including these herbal friends in your self-care regimen.

Holistic wellness goes beyond pain relief. While prompt pain alleviation and inflammatory control are crucial, we'll also stress how important it is to deal with the underlying causes of discomfort. You'll not only reduce symptoms by taking a holistic approach to well-being, but you'll also promote general health and energy.

You'll learn about the tremendous potential of herbs to provide solace and support as you embark on this road of quick pain relief and inflammation control. Come along as we investigate the natural routes to health, led by the knowledge of the plant world and the restorative power of nature.

5.3 Making Homemade Herbal First Aid Kits for Different Situations.

We dig into the useful and empowering chore of creating handmade herbal first aid kits customized to various scenarios in this section of the chapter. These kits will become your trusted allies, prepared to provide natural cures for a variety of frequent illnesses and crises.

- The following items should be included in every first aid kit: Start with comprehending the essential elements of a complete first aid kit. We'll talk about the basic components of any kit, such as bandages, scissors, tweezers, and antiseptics. These are the fundamental components that may be used to incorporate herbal therapies.

- Choosing Herbs for Particular Situations: Different herbal friends are required for various circumstances. We'll walk you through the process of choosing herbs by the kinds of wounds or illnesses you're likely to experience. You will learn to choose the herbs that are most suited for the circumstance, whether it be wounds, bug bites, headaches, or intestinal problems.

- Tinctures, salves, and Other Herbal Preparations for the Kit: It's satisfying to create natural treatments for your first aid box. We'll show you how to make tinctures, salves, balms, and infused oils, as well as how to prepare and package a variety of herbal treatments. You may keep these preparations easily in your kit for quick access.

- Labels and Categories for Effective Kit Organization: You can locate everything you need quickly with a well-organized first aid bag, particularly in an emergency. Learn how to accurately label and classify your herbal treatments. Your emergency response is streamlined by this organization.

- Treating Common Illnesses: From Colds to Cuts: Your first aid pack may be used to manage routine medical issues as well as sudden injuries. We'll discuss the best ways to use herbs that help treat common ailments including colds, headaches, dyspepsia, and small wounds. You'll be ready for both the anticipated and unforeseen with your gear nearby.

- On-the-Go Herbal Support: Travel-Friendly Kits: There are always going to be little mistakes while traveling. Learn how to make portable, compact first aid kits that you can take on travels. No matter where you are in the globe, these kits provide you with the comfort of herbal support.

- Developing Self-Reliance: Belief in Herbal Remedies: Making your herbal first aid kits is a significant step toward independence and natural health. These kits not only provide practical solutions but also give you faith in your capacity to handle medical emergencies successfully.

- The Benefits of Herbal First Aid: Promoting Health Among Others: For friends and family, homemade herbal first aid kits are thoughtful and significant presents. We'll go through how to design kits that are tailored to certain people or circumstances to promote a healthy culture in your neighborhood.

By assembling individualized herbal first aid kits, you'll not only put together supplies for emergency treatment but also foster a closer relationship with the therapeutic potential of herbs. Join us as we set out on this path of readiness and empowerment, aided by the healing powers of nature and the fundamentals of herbalism.

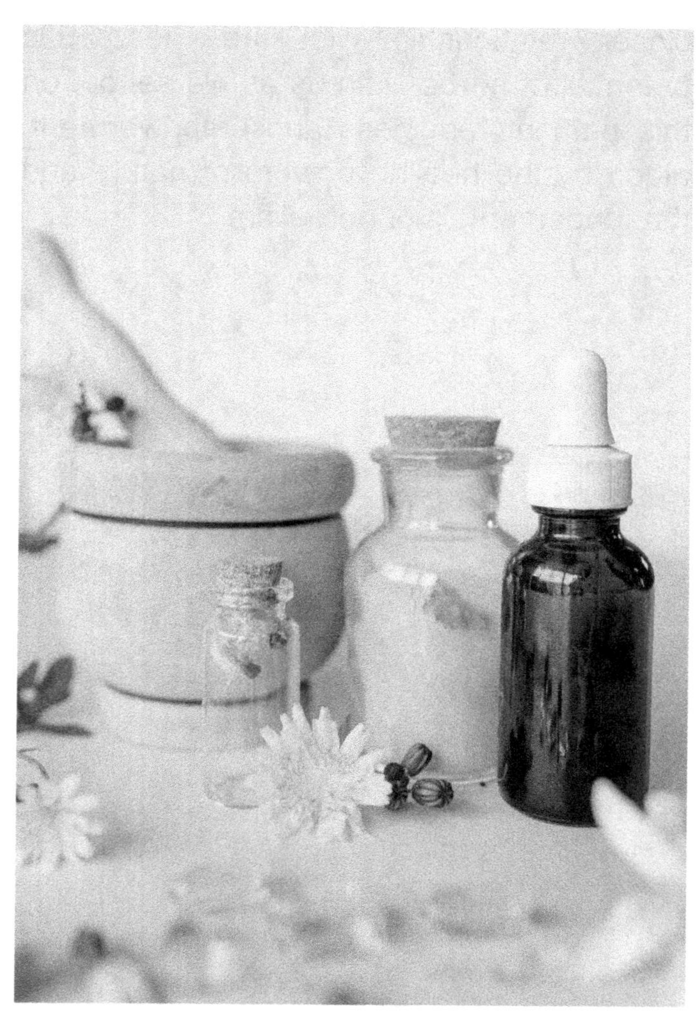

CHAPTER SIX: Respiratory Health and Beyond

6.1 Herbs to Strengthen Lung Health: Respiratory Infections

We move our attention in this chapter to the crucial area of respiratory health, which is a cornerstone of general well-being. We'll look at the powerful herbs that promote respiratory health, support the functioning of the respiratory system, and relieve common respiratory illnesses.

- A Complex Network for Understanding the Respiratory System: Our body's ability to absorb oxygen and eliminate waste is largely dependent on the respiratory system. We'll dig into the complex network of the lungs, bronchi, and airways to comprehend how crucial it is to keep them functioning at their best for general health.

- Herbal Treatments for Respiratory Infections and Their Effects: The ordinary cold and more serious illnesses may both be caused by respiratory infections. Learn how herbs may help you specifically by reducing your symptoms, increasing your immune system, and treating the root causes of illnesses.

- Strengthening defense mechanisms using herbs for immune support: A strong immune system is essential for maintaining respiratory health. Learn about the plants that help the immune system, from elderberry's antiviral qualities to echinacea's immune-modulating benefits. The body's defenses against respiratory infections may be strengthened with the use of these herbs.

- Herbs to Calm Coughs and Clear the Airways: Herbs provide all-natural remedies for coughs and congestion, which may be uncomfortable. Herbs like mullein, thyme, and marshmallow root, each having a special capacity to calm inflamed airways and encourage healthy expectations, will be introduced to you.

- Making Formulas for Respiratory Support: Teas, Syrups, and Steam: Learn how to prepare calming teas, reassuring syrups, and healing steam mixtures with herbs. These remedies may treat a variety of respiratory symptoms, such as chest congestion and scratchy throats, right away and help the body recuperate.

- Utilizing Respiratory Herbs in Daily Life: Preventive Strategies: When it comes to respiratory health, prevention is just as important as treating the symptoms. To preserve lung health and lower the risk of infections, learn how to include respiratory herbs into your daily routine. We'll help you develop a proactive mindset by recommending immune-boosting drinks and aromatherapy techniques.

6.1.1 Navigating Herbal Respiratory Support: Dosage and Duration

To get the results you want from herbal medicines, you must know the right dose and how long to take them. We'll go through how to calculate the ideal dosages of herbs and how to modify the dose following each person's requirements. Potential interactions and safety issues will also be addressed.

Wellness for the Whole Respiratory System: Beyond Herbal Interventions
While herbs are a great aid, lifestyle choices also have an impact on respiratory health. We'll look at how diet, water, exercise, and stress reduction affect our overall respiratory health. You may improve your lung health in many ways by taking a comprehensive approach.

You'll have a clearer understanding of the function that plants play in improving lung health as a result of this investigation into herbs for respiratory illnesses. Join us as we explore the realm of herbal respiratory support, inspired by the wisdom of nature and the quest for inner wellness.

6.2 The Breath of Life: Allergic Remedy and Adjunctive Procedures

We go into the topic of allergy relief and supporting measures for the best possible respiratory health in this section of the chapter. Learn how herbs may help you manage your allergies and give comfort, enabling you to breathe easily and fully appreciate life.

6.2.1 Herbal Insights: Understanding Allergies and Their Effect

Allergies may have a substantial impact on respiratory health and can be more than simply a seasonal annoyance. Understanding how the body's immunological response may cause symptoms like congestion, sneezing, and itching eyes will help us better understand the processes behind allergies.

- Herbs for Allergy Relief: Natural Pain Reliever: Learn more about the herbal allies that may help with allergy problems. We'll introduce you to plants that might lessen allergy pain, from butterbur's possible antihistamine capabilities to stinging nettle's anti-inflammatory benefits.

- Supporting Herbs and Tonics for the Respiratory System: Learn about the nutritious herbs that promote the respiratory system's general health. We'll talk about herbs that may support the lungs and keep them functioning at their best, such as licorice, elecampane, and astragalus.

- Making Formulations for Allergies: Teas, Tinctures, and More: Learn how to make herbal remedies that are particularly intended to treat allergies. We'll show you how to make herbal teas, tinctures, and other concoctions that work in concert with one another. These formulas may reduce symptoms and regulate immunological responses.

- Lifestyle Strategies for Including Herbal Support in Daily Activities: In addition to natural therapies, lifestyle choices are also important in treating allergies. We'll look at how diet, hydration, stress reduction, and environmental changes may all help to lessen allergy symptoms. You'll increase the efficacy of herbal assistance by adopting a comprehensive strategy.

- Building resilience is one of the long-term allergy management strategies. Building resilience to lessen the body's reaction is an important component of managing allergies in addition to treating the symptoms. We'll talk about methods for managing allergies over the long term, such as immune-suppressing herbs and healthy lifestyle habits.

- Herbal solutions that are tailored using individualized approaches: Allergies affect each individual differently. Learn how to tailor herbal remedies to suit specific requirements and sensitivity levels. You may maximize the efficiency of your allergy treatment techniques by customizing herbal therapies.

- Beyond allergy relief, holistic respiratory wellness entails: We will highlight the significance of total wellness even if allergy alleviation is a critical component of respiratory health. You may create long-lasting lung health by adopting holistic respiratory wellness that goes beyond allergy season.

You will acquire the skills to control allergies and breathe more easily via this investigation of allergy relief and supporting measures. Join us as we explore natural cures from nature and the desire for a life full of energy and ease as we explore the world of herbal assistance for respiratory health.

6.3   Natural   Solutions   for Respiratory Wellness Balancing

We explore how herbs may help maintain balance and harmony within the respiratory system in this portion of the chapter as we go further into the holistic approach to respiratory health. Learn about the beneficial interactions between herbs that support lung health and general well-being.

A Comprehensive View of the Holistic Approach to Respiratory Wellness
Beyond only the physical self, holistic health also takes into account one's emotions, thoughts, and spirituality. We'll talk about how an all-encompassing strategy for respiratory wellness promotes a greater feeling of balance by taking into account all aspects of health.

6.3.1 The following herbs strengthen and tonify the lungs:

Investigate the plants that strengthen and promote resiliency in the lungs by acting as tonics. We'll introduce you to herbs that may assist increase oxygenation, support lung function, and all-around lung health, from lungwort to cordyceps.

- Natural Allies for Relaxation and Deep Breathing: In addition to serving a physiological purpose, breathing opens the door to calm and awareness. Learn how herbs like lemon balm, chamomile, and lavender may assist calm, deep breathing to help you relax and reduce stress.

- Teas and Aromatherapy: Creating Herbal Blends for Respiratory Balance: Discover how to create herbal concoctions that support healthy breathing and general well-being. We'll show you how to make herbal teas and aromatherapy mixes with calming smells to improve your respiratory experience.

- Breathwork and meditation have powerful effects on the mind-body connection: Breathwork and meditation techniques may be used to explore the mind-body relationship. We'll talk about how these techniques may improve lung function, control breathing patterns, and promote inner peace.

- Enhancing Respiratory Health via Exercise and Movement: The health of your respiratory system depends on physical exercise. We'll look at how using herbs in addition to regular physical activity may improve oxygenation, circulation, and lung health. Learn which herbs may improve your active lifestyle.

6.3.2 Emotional Wellness: Building Resilience and Inner Balance:

Respiratory health and emotions are closely related. We'll explore how herbs like passionflower and hawthorn may help manage stress, anxiety, and emotional imbalances that may affect breathing as we dig into the emotional side of lung health.

Wellness for the Whole Respiratory System: The Journey Within
By adopting a comprehensive strategy for respiratory health, you set out on a journey that takes into account your physical, emotional, mental, and spiritual well-being. Herbs and attentive techniques may work together harmoniously to help you breathe with balance and vigor.

Join us as we investigate the fascinating relationship between herbs, breath, and overall health. Through this investigation, you'll learn how natural cures may enhance your overall living by promoting a sense of harmony and inner radiance in addition to supporting lung health.

CHAPTER SEVEN: Digestive Wellness: From Garden to Gut

7.1 Herbal Allies for Gut Health: Unraveling Digestive Disorders

This chapter takes us on a tour into the complex realm of digestive wellness, where gut health is crucial to overall well-being. We'll explore the world of digestive issues and introduce you to herbal friends that help rebalance the body and enhance intestinal health.

7.1.1 The Contribution of Digestive Health to General Wellness: A Holistic View:

The digestive tract is vital to health and affects many internal processes in addition to its role in breaking down food. We'll look at how immunity, mental health, and energy levels are all impacted by intestinal health.

7.1.2 Herbal Treatments for Common Digestive Disorders and Their Effects

Indigestion, bloating, and other more complicated digestive issues may cause everyday disruptions. Learn how using herbs may help treat the underlying causes of many conditions, alleviate symptoms, and promote the body's healing mechanisms.

- Herbs for Soothing and Comforting the Digestive System: Discover the herbs that help soothe pain and encourage gastrointestinal ease. We'll introduce you to herbs that help ease typical digestive concerns, such as the anti-nausea benefits of ginger and the calming qualities of peppermint.

- Herbal Prebiotics and Probiotics Balance the Gut Microbiota: For good digestion and general well-being, a healthy gut microbiome is essential. Learning how to include probiotic-rich herbs that support a varied microbial balance and supplying prebiotic fibers that feed beneficial bacteria are two ways that herbs may improve gut health.

- Making Formulas for Digestive Support: Teas, Infusions, and Bitters: Learn how to include herbs into formulations that assist digestion and benefit many elements of gut health. We'll show you how to make teas, infusions, and bitters that aid in digestion, enhance nutrient absorption, and soothe pain.

- Beyond Meals: Including Herbs in Digestive Lifestyle Habits: It's not simply what you eat that affects your digestive health; it's also how you live. Learn how to include herbs into routines that support healthy digestion, such as movement, breathing exercises, and mindfulness.

- Finding the Ideal Balance for Digestive Health: Dosage and

Duration: For digestive well-being, it's crucial to comprehend the right herbal remedy dose and length. We'll go through how to customize herbal therapies based on the patient's unique requirements to provide successful and secure results.

- Wellness of the Digestive System: Nourishing Body and Soul: You may nourish both your physical and emotional well-being by adopting a holistic approach to digestive health. We'll look at how herbs may promote emotional harmony, stress reduction, and a healthy relationship with food.

You'll have a better knowledge of the significant function that herbs play in enhancing digestion and general vigor as a result of this investigation into digestive issues and herbal allies for gut health. Join us as we explore the world of digestive health, inspired by plant knowledge and the desire for a body and spirit that are both well-nourished.

7.2 Herbs for Bloating, Indigestion, and Other Digestive Issues

We explore how herbs might provide comfort and support for common problems including indigestion, bloating, and more in this chapter's section on particular digestive concerns. You can traverse digestive difficulties with confidence if you are aware of the qualities of these plants.

7.2.1 The Complexity of Indigestion and Bloating: Understanding Digestive Challenges

The most frequent digestive symptoms, including indigestion and bloating, may negatively impact everyday comfort and well-being. We'll examine the underlying causes of these difficulties and learn how stress, nutrition, and lifestyle may affect them.

- Calming the Digestive Fire: Herbal Allies for Indigestion Relief: Investigate the plants that help alleviate and relax gastrointestinal distress. We'll introduce you to herbs that may help with indigestion relief and encourage a feeling of comfort, from chamomile's anti-inflammatory benefits to fennel's carminative characteristics.

- Using Digestive Bitters and Carminatives to Reduce Bloating: Although bloating may be annoying, there are herbal remedies available. Learn how digestive bitters and carminative herbs help improve bloating, encourage gas release, and improve digestion. We'll show you how to include these herbs in your everyday regimen.

- Supporting enzymes and nutrient absorption using herbs for optimal digestion: In addition to preventing pain, effective nutrition absorption is another goal of optimal digestion. Discover how herbs such as gentian and ginger may promote the release of digestive enzymes, help in nutrient absorption, and improve general well-being.

- Teas, tinctures, and aromatherapy for the creation of customized digestive formulas: Making custom herbal remedies enables you to create treatments that are tailored to your unique digestion requirements. We'll look at how to make tinctures, teas, and aromatherapy mixtures that treat bloating, indigestion, and other problems.

- Beyond herbal remedies: Lifestyle Strategies for Digestive Wellness: Herbs are effective friends, but lifestyle choices are also very important for digestive health. Examine how stress reduction, mindful eating, and hydration promote healthy digestion and increase the efficacy of herbal assistance.

7.2.2 Navigating Herbal Solutions for Digestive Challenges: Dosage and Duration

To get the results you want from herbal medicines, you must know the right dose and how long to take them. We'll go through how to calculate the ideal dosages of herbs and how to modify the dose by each person's requirements. Potential interactions and safety issues will also be addressed.

- Integrative digestive wellness: embracing harmony and balance: Keep in mind that holistic well-being includes not just physical health but also emotional and mental well-being when you use herbs to address digestive issues. You may attain intestinal harmony by cultivating a healthy connection with food and feeding your complete self.

You'll learn important things about how nature's cures may provide comfort and support digestive health via this investigation of herbs for indigestion, bloating, and other issues. Join us as we explore the world of digestive support, aided by the knowledge of herbs and the desire to live in harmony with our bodies.

7.3 Using herbal remedies to nourish the digestive system

We go into the idea of feeding the digestive tract using herbal remedies in this section of the chapter. Learn how herbs may help the complex processes of digestion and absorption to give vital nutrients, encourage gut health, and contribute to overall well-being.

7.3.1. Understanding Digestive Nourishment: Nutrient Intake's Importance

Digestion involves more than simply breaking down food; it also involves removing essential elements for health and energy. We'll look at how herbs may provide the critical vitamins, minerals, and chemicals the digestive system needs to work at its best.

- Using herbs as nutrient-dense foods is a healthy alternative: A broad variety of vitamins, minerals, and antioxidants may be found in many herbs, making them nutritional powerhouses. We'll show you how to include nettles, dandelion greens, and chickweed into meals and liquids for improved digestive hydration.

- Supporting the Microbiota and Gut Lining with Herbs: For optimal digestion and nutritional absorption, a healthy gut lining and bacteria are necessary. Learn how the calming and nourishing qualities of plants like marshmallow root, slippery elm, and licorice may improve intestinal health.

- Strengthening digestive function using herbal tonics for digestive vitality: Learn more about the idea of herbal tonics that energize and support the digestive system. We'll introduce you to a wide variety of herbs that support vitality and well-being, ranging from astringent herbs that stimulate digestive fluids to adaptogens that improve stress resistance.

7.3.2 Formulating Herbal Tonics and Elixirs: Digestive Nourishing Blends:

Learn how to make herbal elixirs and tonics that provide a concentrated dose of gastrointestinal hydration. We'll help you create concoctions that include nutrient-rich herbs with other supporting components to boost the overall effectiveness of these treatments.

- Adding Herbs to Culinary Creations: Combining Flavor and Wellness: Herbs may enhance the taste and nutritional content of your meals in addition to being used in treatments. Learn how to use herbs in your cooking to enhance the flavor and health benefits of your food.

- Navigating Herbal Digestive Nourishment: Dosage and Duration: To get the best benefits, it is essential to comprehend the right herbal dose and time for digestion nutrition. To optimize the advantages of these treatments, we'll provide you with advice on how to include them in your routine.

- Integrative Digestive Wellness: Promoting Balance and Nourishment: You're building a closer relationship with your body's requirements and advancing general well-being by supporting your digestive system with herbal remedies. Accept a holistic approach to digestive health that takes into account not just the foods you eat but also how you fuel your complete self.

You will learn about the potent ways that herbs may boost gut health and general energy via this investigation of supporting the digestive system using herbal remedies. Come along with us as we explore the realm of digestive health, led by the knowledge of nature's cures and the desire for a well-fed body.

CHAPTER EIGHT: Skin Soothing and Restoration

8.1 The Skin-Healing Arsenal: Natural Treatments for Skin Disorders

In this chapter, we examine the topic of skin health and renewal, an area in which herbs are very important for calming and repairing the skin. We'll explore the herbal remedies that may help relieve pain and improve skin health for anything from basic skin irritations to more complicated disorders.

8.1.1 Beyond aesthetics, the significance of skin health is as follows:

Skin serves as more than simply our outside covering; it serves as a barrier of protection and a window into our interior well-being. Understanding how the state of the skin might reflect underlying imbalances will help us to address the significance of skin health in connection to overall well-being.

- Skin Disorders and Their Effects: Herbal Treatments: Dryness, rashes, or more severe skin disorders may make people feel uncomfortable and insecure. Learn how herbs may provide relief by treating the underlying causes of skin problems and offering kind and efficient remedies.

- Herbs that Reduce Itching and Inflammation and Soothe Skin Irritations include: Investigate the plants that may make skin irritations less painful. We'll introduce you to herbs that help relieve itching, redness, and inflammation, from calendula's anti-inflammatory benefits to chamomile's calming characteristics.

8.1.2 Using Herbal Infusions and Oils to Nourish and Hydrate Skin

Learn to make herbal oils and infusions that may moisturize and nourish the skin to the core. We'll talk about plants that may improve skin health and bring back their natural brightness, such as lavender, rose, and comfrey.

- Topical Solutions for Restoration: Herbal Skin Salve and Balm Formulation: Learn how to turn herbs into topical treatments that promote skin repair. We'll show you how to make herbal salves and balms that may be administered directly to affected regions, acting as a barrier and hastening the healing process.

- Beyond Remedies: Including Skin-Friendly Herbs in Personal Care: Skin health involves adopting a comprehensive approach to personal care as well as using specialized treatments. Learn how to use mild cleansers and nourishing masks that include skin-friendly herbs in your daily regimen.

8.1.3 Navigating Herbal Solutions for Skin Health: Dosage and Duration

To get the results you want from herbal medicines, you must know the right dose and how long to take them. We'll go through how to calculate the ideal dosages of herbs and how to modify the dose by each person's requirements. Potential interactions and safety issues will also be addressed.

- Holistic Skin Wellness: Promoting Radiance from the Inside Out: As you explore the realm of herbal treatments for skin issues, keep in mind that good skin well-being extends beyond simple maintenance. You'll exude health from the inside out if you adopt a holistic strategy that takes into account diet, hydration, stress management, and emotional well-being.

You will learn important information about the significant ways that herbs may assist skin health and renewal via this investigation of herbal treatments for skin disorders. Join us as we explore the world of skin calming and restoration, led by the knowledge of natural cures and the desire for healthy, bright skin.

8.2 Plant-Based Treatments for Irritations and Eruptions

In this Section, we go further into the area of employing plant-based therapies to soothe skin eruptions and irritations. Learn how herbs may provide relief from itchiness, redness, and irritation so you can develop healthy, peaceful skin.

8.2.1 Understanding Skin Eruptions and Irritations: Contributing Factors and Treatment Options

Allergies, environmental triggers, stress, and other factors may all cause skin irritations and breakouts. We'll examine the root causes of these problems and how the body's reactions produce pain.

- The following are some natural remedies for calming irritated skin: Learn about a variety of herbs that may cool and reduce inflammation to calm sensitive skin. We'll introduce you to herbs that help soothe and calm sensitive regions, from chamomile's mild relief to aloe vera's moisturizing properties.

- Bath blends and compresses: Using Herbal Infusions for Skin Relief: Discover how to use herbal infusions to make calming bath mixes and compresses. Through these treatments, herbs may directly soothe sensitive skin conditions and improve the health of the whole skin surface.

- Making Herbal-Infused Oils for the Skin: Nourishment and Restoration: Learn the trade of creating herbal-infused oils that are designed to soothe the skin. We'll show you how to make oils infused with plants that have been picked for their capacity to hydrate, mend, and revitalize the skin, including lavender, calendula, and chamomile.

8.2.2 Topical Comfort: Creating Calming Skin Salves and Creams

Discover the world of herbal creams and salves created to provide specific relief for sensitive skin. Learn how to make formulations that blend different herbs with nourishing oils and butter to produce a layer that is both therapeutic and protective.

- Examining Herbal Anti-Itch Treatments: Controlling the Necessity to Scratch: Herbs provide ways to control the need to scratch, which may be irritating if you have itchy skin. We'll introduce you to plants that may soothe itching and lessen the chance of developing more irritation, from witch hazel to plantain.

- Applying herbal remedies for skin relief: Dosage and Time: For desired results, it is crucial to know how to administer herbal skin treatment remedies. We'll go through how to choose the best application techniques and how to modify treatments according to patient requirements.

- Holistic Skin Wellness: Developing Inner Calm and Comfort: Keep in mind that holistic skin health goes beyond topical medications as you research plant-based solutions for soothing skin breakouts and irritated skin. You may improve the efficiency of herbal therapies by addressing possible internal causes and adopting stress-reduction techniques.

You will learn useful techniques to support skin comfort and wellness via this investigation of herbal treatments for skin eruptions and irritants. Join us as we explore the world of plant-based remedies, led by the knowledge of herbs and the desire for peaceful, glowing skin.

8.3 Maintain the Radiance of Your Skin: Herbal Beauty and Wellness

This section of the chapter explores the idea of enhancing the brightness of your skin via the use of herbal beauty and health treatments. Investigate how herbs may improve the radiance of your skin, enhancing not just its outside beauty but also its inner vigor and well-being.

8.3.1 Beauty Beyond Surface: Embracing the Idea of Radiant Skin

Not only does radiant skin look good, but it also reflects good health, vigor, and self-care. We'll talk about the holistic approach to beauty and how using herbs may improve one's inner and outer attractiveness.

- Nourishment and Vitality: Herbal Allies for Increasing Skin's Natural Glow: Learn about herbs that may revitalize and nourish the layers of your skin to boost its natural radiance. We'll introduce you to herbs that support radiant and healthy skin, from hibiscus' brightening characteristics to rosehips' abundant antioxidant content.

- Developing Self-Care Rituals: Making Herbal Facial Steams and Masks: Discover how to prepare nutritious and opulent herbal face steams and masks. These procedures may help to open pores, nourish the skin with beneficial herbs, and provide brief periods of rest and renewal.

- Hydrosols and Toners Infused with Herbs to Balance and Refresh the Skin: Discover the world of hydrosols and toners with herbal infusions to help balance and refresh the skin. We'll help you create formulas that moisturize, tone, and give your skin a little nutritional boost, leaving it feeling refreshed.

- Making Deep Nourishment and Renewal Herbal Infused Serums and Elixirs: Explore the process of creating herbal-infused serums and elixirs that provide the skin with intense nutrition and rejuvenation. Learn how to build formulas that penetrate deeply and stimulate cellular renewal by combining oils infused with strong botanicals.

- Investigating Herbal Bath Soaks: Wellness for the Body and Soul: Discover the advantages of herbal bath soaks that enhance not only the health of your skin but also your whole well-being. Discover how to make opulent bath routines that use herbs, salts, and fragrant essential oils for a whole sense of relaxation.

- Applying Herbal Beauty and Wellness Practices: Dosage and

Duration: For desired results, it is crucial to know how to implement herbal beauty and health techniques. We'll go through how to include these techniques into your self-care regimen so that you may enjoy both effectiveness and nurturing.

A journey of self-love and care, holistic skin wellness
Keep in mind that the path is one of self-love and care as you cultivate the brightness of your skin via herbal beauty and health practices. By adopting holistic skin health, you'll not only improve your outward beauty but also foster a stronger sense of self-awareness.

You'll learn how herbs may improve your self-care regimen and improve the vibrancy of your skin via this investigation of herbal beauty and wellness techniques. Join us as we explore the realm of herbal radiance, inspired by the beauty and inner harmony that comes from using nature's cures.

PART FIVE: Making Herbal Remedies

CHAPTER NINE: Mastering Herbal Formulas

9.1 Creating potent herbal blends: The Art of Synergy

This chapter delves into the complex process of creating herbal concoctions that harness the power of synergy—the combined effects of properly chosen plants acting in unison. Learn how to combine herbs to increase their medicinal value and produce cures that are more effective than the sum of their parts.

9.1.1 Herbs in Concert: Understanding the Power of Synergy

The hidden component that elevates herbal remedies to extraordinary status is synergy. We'll look at the idea of synergy to see how several herbs may complement one another's effects and provide a well-rounded and effective treatment.

- Matching actions and energies will help you choose herbs for maximum synergy: The selection of herbs that complement each other's activities and energies is the first step in creating potent herbal blends. Learn how to choose herbs that treat several facets of an illness to promote a holistic and diverse healing process.

- Choosing the Right Ingredients for Herbal Formulas to Get the Best Results: Learn how to balance herbal elements in a mix to get the results you want. We'll talk about the ratio of herbs, and doses, and how to modify formulas to unique requirements and sensitivities.

- Herbal Remedies for Particular Illnesses: Customized Treatments: Using the information from earlier chapters, investigate the creation of herbal remedies for certain diseases. Whether it's digestive support, skin calming, or respiratory wellness, we'll help you create potent mixes that address specific health issues.

- The Function of Herbal Energetics: Harmonizing the Yin and Yang: You may use knowledge of herbal energetics to create formulae that balance the body's pH by determining if a plant is dampening or drying, warming or cooling, etc. Learn how to use these ideas to modify formulae to fit each person's constitution.

- Personalized Medicine: Customizing Herbal Blends for Individual Needs: The way the body reacts to herbal treatments varies from person to person. We'll look at how to alter herbal mixtures according to a person's requirements, taking into consideration things like age, constitution, and the existence of other medical issues.

- Making Herbal Formulas for Various Preparations, including Teas, Tinctures, and More: Learn how to modify your herbal formulations for various forms of application, including teas, tinctures, salves, and more. You may choose the preparation technique that will provide the results you want since each one comes with special advantages and delivery options.

9.1.2 How to Create Effective Herbal Blends: Dosage and Duration

To get the best benefits from herbal formulae, you must be aware of the right dose and time frame. We'll provide instructions on how to choose doses depending on unique circumstances and how to modify therapies over time.

- Holistic herbal remedies: fusing nature's knowledge: You may access the essence of nature's knowledge and the amazing synergy that herbs give by developing the skill of creating potent herbal mixes. You'll produce treatments via this fusion that connect with the body's intrinsic ability to heal and maintain balance.

You'll learn how to make strong and individualized treatments by learning about the synergy principle and creating herbal mixtures that work. Join us as we explore the world of herbal formulations in more detail, led by the complex dance of interacting plants.

9.2 Creating Blends for Particular Health Issues

In this chapter's section, we go further into the process of creating herbal concoctions that are designed to address certain health issues. You may develop specialized treatments that address a variety of conditions and promote holistic well-being by comprehending the special qualities of herbs and how they interact.

9.2.1 Herbal Synergy's Science Revealed: A Deeper Exploration

Explore the science of herbal synergy to learn how the interaction of different substances in herbs may enhance their benefits. Learn how certain herbs might cooperate to address various facets of a health condition.

- Making Respiratory Support Formulas to Facilitate Comfort and Breathing: Learn how to create herbal concoctions that assist breathing and promote the best possible lung health and breathing comfort. Discover how to choose herbs that support general respiratory health, relieve inflammation, and remove congestion.

9.2.2 Digestive Harmony Formulas: Promoting Gut Wellness and Digestion

Explore the world of herbal combinations that may help you with indigestion, bloating, and pain. Find out which plants may help you digest food properly, maintain a healthy gut microbiome, and reduce inflammation.

- Blends for Skin Healing: Increasing Radiance and Comfort: Discover the world of herbal concoctions created to hydrate and revive the health and brightness of the skin. Find out how to blend herbs that treat a variety of skin disorders, reduce inflammation, and encourage cellular regeneration.

- Herbs for Mind and Mood Support: Emotional Well-Being Formulas: Learn how to create herbal mixtures that can enhance emotional health. Investigate the plants that have soothing effects, aid in stress management, and promote mental balance and harmony.

- Women's Health Formulas: Addressing Comfort and Hormonal Balance: Explore the development of herbal concoctions that promote women's health, including hormone imbalances, menstruation pain, and other associated issues. Discover how to choose plants that support balanced hormones and general health.

- Developing Herbal Supplements for Daily Wellness: A Preventive Approach: Learn how to create herbal mixes for daily well-being using a preventative healthcare approach. Learn about herbs that may be used in everyday routines to improve resilience, vigor, and immunity.

- Making Targeted Herbal Blends: Dosage and Duration: To acquire the intended outcomes from specific herbal mixes, it is crucial to understand the right dose and time.

We'll go through how to adjust doses to suit each person's demands and particular health issues while still guaranteeing safety.

- Integrative herbal remedies: a tapestry of wellness: You may create mixes to address certain health issues, creating a tapestry of well-being that includes the body and the spirit. You may make remedies that strongly connect with the body's intrinsic ability for healing by combining herbs in a way that promotes harmony.

You will learn the skills to treat a variety of illnesses and encourage holistic well-being via this investigation of creating blends for certain health issues. Come explore the artistry of making precise medicines with us as we are inspired by the complex dance of herbs and the quest for total wellness and vitality.

9.3 A Comprehensive Examination of Combination Herbal Treatments

In this section of the chapter, we go further into the world of combination herbal treatments and examine the subtleties of combining various plants to produce effective and all-encompassing cures. Learn the skill of harmonizing diverse qualities and energies to handle complicated health issues and get the best outcomes.

9.3.1 A multifaceted approach to "Unlocking the Potential of Combination Remedies"

Combination herbal treatments provide a multifaceted approach to healing where the potent effects of many plants work together. We'll look at how several herbs might be picked to work in harmony with one another and provide a comprehensive remedy.

- Increasing defenses and resilience while developing immune-boosting formulas: Investigate the development of combination medications that promote immunological health. Learn how to choose immune-boosting plants that cooperate to bolster the body's defenses and encourage general health.

- Formulas for balancing hormonal harmony that support reproductive health: Learn the subtleties of creating blends of medications that promote reproductive health and hormonal balance. Discover how to choose plants that balance the endocrine system and reduce menstruation pain.

- Herbs for Emotional Balance and Cognitive Function: Mind-Body Wellness Blends: Investigate the realm of complementary treatments for mind-body wellbeing. Learn how to include herbs that support emotional balance and mental clarity into mixes that treat stress, anxiety, and cognitive function.

9.3.2 Combinations for Digestive Comfort: Promoting Gut Health

Recognize the technique of creating mixture cures for gastrointestinal ease. Discover the best ways to mix herbs that address different elements of digestion, microbial balance, and gut integrity.

- Formulas for Optimal Skin Health: Holistic Approaches to Radiance: Investigate the development of fusion treatments that encourage ideal skin health. Learn how to choose herbs that complement one another to treat skin issues, promote hydration, and improve the skin's brightness.

- Navigating Combination Herbal Remedies: Dosage and Duration: To get the results you want from a combination herbal remedy, you must know the right dose and time. We'll go through how to alter doses according to the number of herbs in the mix and how to make sure it's harmonious and efficient.

- Creating Holistic Balance and Wellness with Herbal Medicine: Holistic Herbal Mastery: You are mastering the art of holistic balance and well-being by learning the intricate details of herbal combinations. You'll create treatments that respect the complexities of the human body and its intrinsic ability to heal by fusing carefully chosen herbs.

You'll learn more about the tremendous effects that many herbs acting synergistically may have on health and well-being via this investigation of herbal combinations. Join us as we explore the world of herbal formulations more thoroughly, led by the complex dance of the plants and the desire for complete wellness and vitality.

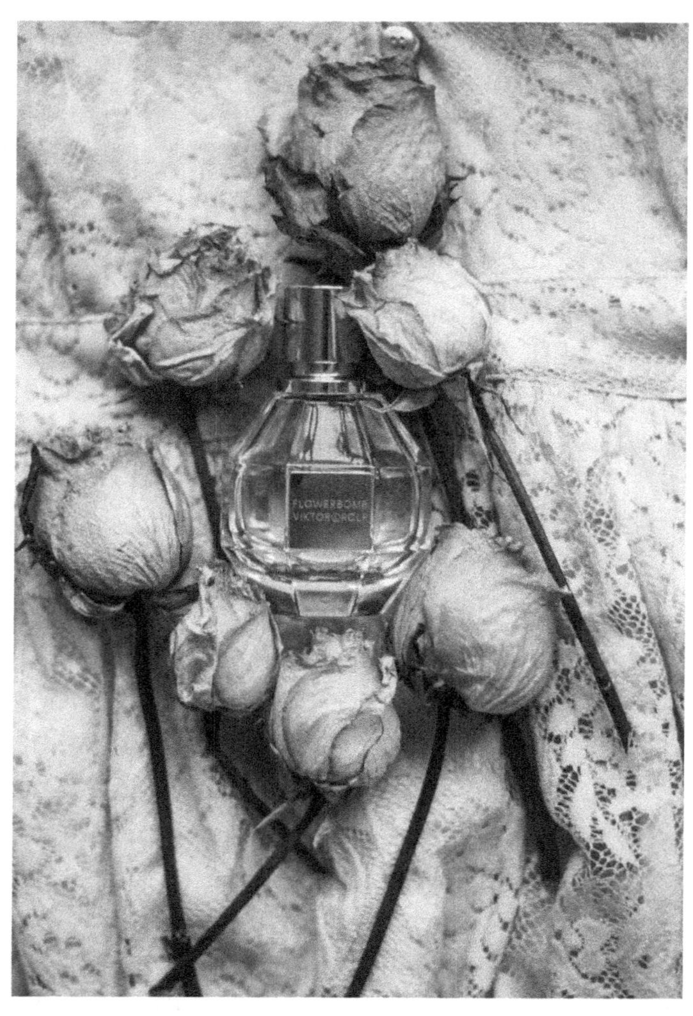
FLOWERBOMB
VIKTOR&ROLF

CHAPTER TEN: Sustainable Herbal Practice

10.1 Growing Herbs at Home in Your Healing Garden

In this chapter, we examine the delightful activity of creating your herb-filled healing garden. Learn about the benefits of cultivating herbs at home and how to build a supportive space that will help you feel profoundly connected to nature's healing powers.

10.1.1 Embracing Nature's Wisdom: The Garden as a Healing Sanctuary

More than simply a collection of plants, a healing garden is a haven that fosters your relationship with nature and provides a place for solace and introspection. We'll talk about how spending time in your garden may be soothing and how deeply plants and well-being are connected.

- Choosing Herbs for Your Healing Garden: Goals and Intentions: Learn about the selection process for the herbs you want to grow in your healing garden. Learn how to choose herbs that support your health objectives, whether you're growing them for specialized therapeutic purposes, delicious culinary uses, or aesthetic beauty.

- Layout, Soil, and Sunlight in Garden Design: Learn the components of creating a flourishing healing garden. We'll go through issues like garden design, soil preparation, and the best sunlight exposure to create a space where herbs may thrive and provide their full therapeutic potential.

- Watering, pruning, and harvesting are all aspects of taking care of your herbal allies: Learn how to take good care of your herbal companions at all stages of their development. You'll learn tips for managing a flourishing garden, from watering procedures that stimulate healthy development to pruning methods that boost vitality.

- Herbs should be harvested with the purpose to respect the plant's gift: Examine the importance of gathering herbs with awareness and purpose. Learn the best times to harvest various plant components, as well as how to retain their potency via drying and storage methods.

10.1.2 Creating Herbal Reflection Spaces: Developing the Mind and Spirit

Learn how to create an area for contemplation and meditation in your healing garden. Discover how spending time with your herbs may promote a feeling of calm and connection, enabling you to access the natural world's healing power.

- Sustainable Gardening Techniques: Cooperating with Nature: Recognize the significance of eco-friendly gardening techniques that put plant and ecosystem health first. Learn about strategies including soil augmentation, companion planting, and eco-friendly insect management.

- Holistic herbal gardening: Promoting Wellness and Balance: You are participating in a holistic activity that promotes your well-being on several levels by tending to your healing garden. You'll encourage a feeling of balance and harmony within yourself and the environment by working in symbiotic interaction with your herbs and the land.

You will learn a lot about the significant relationship between plants and well-being as you explore how to grow your healing garden. Embark on a trip with us as we explore the realm of sustainable herbal practice, inspired by the knowledge of nature's cures and the desire for peaceful cohabitation with the natural world.

10.2 Respecting the Balance of Nature in Wildcrafting

This chapter's last portion delves into the ethical wildcrafting method, a sustainable and ethical technique to gather herbs from their natural environments. Investigate ethical methods for gathering wild plants to protect the future viability of herbal resources and the fragile ecological balance.

The fundamental principle of ethical wildcrafting is respecting nature's abundance.
A profound regard for nature's bounty and the fragile ecosystems that sustain it is the foundation of ethical wildcrafting. We'll talk about the value of conscientious harvesting and the moral concepts that underpin it.

10.2.1 Understanding Plant Ecology: Awareness of and Impact on Ecosystems

Explore the realm of plant ecology to learn how herbs interact with their surroundings and what functions they serve in regional ecosystems. Acquire knowledge about plant identification, population estimation, and place selection for harvesting to reduce ecological effects.

- Harvesting with Care: Guidelines for Responsible Wildcrafting: Investigate rules for ethical wildcrafting that guarantee the survival of plant populations and environments. We'll talk about techniques like leaving no trace and keeping a respectful distance from sensitive regions.

- Gathering for Health and Nutrition: Wildcrafting with Intention: Learn how to go about wildcrafting with purpose, appreciating the worth of the plants you harvest for food and medicine. Discover the value of communicating with plants, expressing your thanks, and developing a mutually beneficial connection.

- Harvesting and processing in harmony using moral methods: Discover the equipment and methods used in ethical wildcrafting to encourage stewardship of the environment and respect for plant life. We'll show you how to cause the least amount of environmental impact possible, from correct harvesting techniques to careful processing.

10.2.2 The Art of Ethical Wildcrafting: A Lifelong Learning Process

The practice of ethical wildcrafting involves ongoing learning and development. We'll talk about how maintaining this practice requires community involvement, education, and information exchange.

- Sustainable Development and Stewardship: Appreciating Nature's Gifts: Being an ethical wildcrafter makes you a custodian of the earth and everything it has to offer. You're helping to preserve plant variety and the health of the ecosystems that support us all by acting with awareness.

You will develop a profound understanding of the interdependence of all life through this investigation of ethical wildcrafting, as well as the part you may play in maintaining the delicate balance of nature. Join us as we set off on a journey of ethical wildcrafting, motivated by the knowledge of respecting and protecting nature, and sustainable herbal practice.

10.3 Environmentally Friendly Methods of Herbal Healing

This section of the chapter delves into environmentally friendly herbal therapy methods that put the health of the environment first and help create a more sustainable future. Investigate ways to integrate eco-friendly activities into your herbal journey so that your attempts to heal coincide with the health of the ecosystem.

10.3.1 The Connection Between Environmental Wellness and Herbal Healing: A Holistic View

Herbal treatments that are eco-friendly acknowledge the connection between environmental health and human health. We'll investigate how using herbal remedies might benefit the environment and our health.

- Sustainable Herb Sourcing: Giving Ethical and Regenerative Suppliers Priority: Learn why it's important to buy herbs from vendors that value moral behavior and environmental sustainability. Learn how to recognize sources that sustain ecosystems and communities and are in line with your environmental beliefs.

- Herbal Footprint Reduction: Minimize Waste and Packaging: Investigate ways to lessen waste and packaging associated with your herbal use. Discover how to get bulk herbs, reuse or recycle herbal containers, and choose environmentally friendly packaging solutions.

- Herbal crafting with zero waste: inventive reuse and considerate production: Find out how to apply zero-waste concepts to your herbal-making projects. Learn innovative methods to reuse resources, reduce the usage of single-use goods, and participate in conscious manufacturing techniques that produce little waste.

- Making decisions that matter for environmentally friendly herbal preparations: Investigate methods that are environmentally sustainable for making herbal remedies such as teas, tinctures, and salves. Learn how to acquire sustainable ingredients, utilize locally grown plants, and use less non-renewable resources.

10.3.2 Herbal Storage and Packaging: Selecting Sustainable Options

Learn how to choose environmentally friendly choices for storing and packing herbs. Investigate recyclable, biodegradable, or reusable materials to make sure your herbal goods adhere to your goal to live an environmentally responsible life.

- Integral Harmony: Harmonizing Individual Healing and Global Well-Being: You are embracing a holistic harmony that goes beyond personal well-being to the health of the earth by using eco-friendly methods for herbal therapy. You're helping to create a more sustainable and balanced world by coordinating your activities with your environmentally aware decisions.

You'll acquire an understanding of how your decisions may have a good effect on the environment while promoting your health via this investigation of environmentally friendly methods for herbal medicine. Join us as we explore the world of environmentally responsible herbal practice, led by the knowledge of sustainable living and the desire for a more livable earth for all creatures.

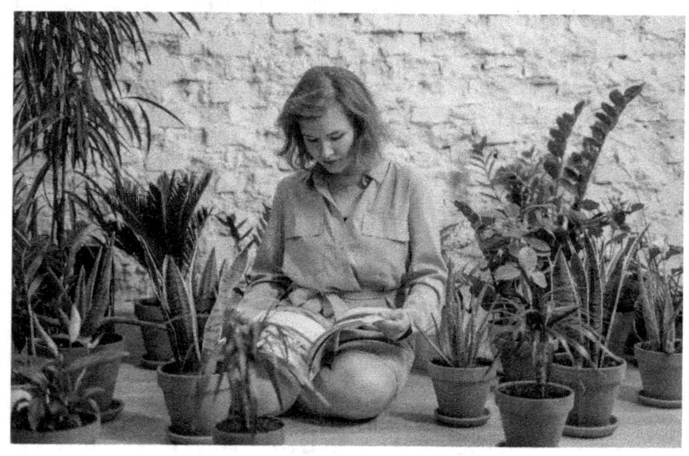

PART FIVE:
Empowerment and Integration

CHAPTER ELEVEN: Combining Herbal Wisdom: Lessons from Three Books

11.1 Bringing Natural and Modern Healing Together: Insights from "Herbal Antibiotics"

We set out on a trip in this chapter to combine the knowledge from the three books we've looked at: "The Modern Herbal Dispensatory," "Herbal Antibiotics," and "Encyclopedia of Herbal Medicine." We start by exploring the revelations and lessons provided by "Herbal Antibiotics," bridging the gap between conventional herbal knowledge and contemporary medical procedures.

11.1.1 Understanding the "Herbal Antibiotics" Paradigm: A New Perspective

By demonstrating the efficacy of plant-based substitutes, "Herbal Antibiotics" challenges the current understanding of antibiotics. We'll look at the idea of herbal antibiotics as a link between conventional medicine and alternative herbal treatments.

- The Strength of Nature's Defenses: Developing Immunity and Resilience: Learn how herbal antibiotics boost the body's natural defenses while improving resilience and immunological function. We'll look at the plants with antibacterial characteristics and how they might improve general health.

- Herbal Allies for Contemporary Challenges: Combating Antibiotic Resistance: Investigate the connections between the lessons learned from "Herbal Antibiotics" and the widespread issue of antibiotic resistance. Discover how using natural medicines may effectively treat bacterial infections while reducing the danger of resistance.

11.2 Integrating Wisdom: Harmonizing with "The Modern Herbal Dispensatory"

We'll go more into the integration of "Herbal Antibiotics" with the ideas from "The Modern Herbal Dispensatory." Examine how herbal antibiotic efficacy may be improved through the art of medicine-making and herbal formulation.

A Balanced Approach to Enhancing Healing Through Holistic Integration
You may establish a way that strikes a balance between the best aspects of conventional and cutting-edge therapeutic techniques by fusing the ideas from "Herbal Antibiotics" with the complete strategy of "The Modern Herbal Dispensatory." You are

given the ability to make well-informed decisions thanks to its integration.

You will have a greater understanding of how herbal knowledge and contemporary treatment techniques work in harmony via this investigation of concepts from "Herbal Antibiotics." Join us as we combine information from many sources to provide you with a comprehensive understanding and the skills you need to take control of your health path.

11.2.1 Making herbal preparations: Advice from "The Modern Herbal Dispensatory"

We now investigate the knowledge provided by "The Modern Herbal Dispensatory" in the context of creating herbal preparations as we continue our integration journey. This information may be combined with the understanding from the previous two volumes to create a complete strategy for using herbs' therapeutic properties.

- Herbal Preparations: The Art and Science of Making Them: Harmonizing Tradition and Modernity: The idea of herbal antibiotics was first given to us in "Herbal Antibiotics," and "The Modern Herbal Dispensatory" gives us the practical information we need to make effective herbal remedies. We'll look at how to create successful cures by blending conventional wisdom with contemporary knowledge.

- Choosing High-Quality Herbs for Best Results: A Fusion of Information: We'll dig into the process of choosing high-quality plants for creating herbal remedies, drawing on the insights of all three volumes. Learn to recognize powerful herbs with antibacterial characteristics so you can include them in different treatments.

11.2.2 Combining Wisdom for Healing: Producing Herbal Extracts and Formulas

Learn how to make herbal tinctures, teas, extracts, and more by using the information provided in all three volumes. Learn how to create well-balanced formulations by studying extraction techniques, dosage issues, and formulation art.

- The holistic method of making medicine: nurturing the mind, body, and spirit: We will investigate how creating herbal preparations may turn into a spiritual activity that nourishes the body, mind, and spirit by combining the ideas of holistic healing and medicine-making. Recognize how intention and awareness play a part in the process.

- A holistic wellness toolkit called "Empowerment through Self-Care": By combining the knowledge from "The Modern Herbal Dispensatory" and other publications, you can assemble your own set of tools for holistic well-being. Learn how to create treatments that address both immediate and long-term health issues, promoting resilience and self-care.

- An Integration of Thoughts: Combining Wisdom for Empowerment: You start a path of empowerment and healing by combining the lessons from all three books. A complete framework for managing your health and well-being is provided by the combination of herbal antibiotics, making remedies, and holistic concepts.

You will learn more about creating herbal preparations and how they fit into the larger framework of herbal medicine via this investigation of "The Modern Herbal Dispensatory." Join us as we continue integrating information, motivated by the aim to provide you with a comprehensive toolset for empowerment and well-being.

11.3 Comprehensive Healing Insights from the "Encyclopedia of Herbal Medicine"

As we go forward on our integration journey, we now dig into the wealth of information offered by the "Encyclopedia of Herbal Medicine." We'll discover a holistic approach to herbal health and well-being by fusing the knowledge from this comprehensive resource with the understanding from the previous two volumes.

11.3.1 A Multifaceted View of the Herbal Treasure Chest in the Encyclopedia

The "Encyclopedia of Herbal Medicine" provides a wide variety of herbs and treatments for different diseases. We'll look at how this source's information, together with the lessons from the other books, offers a holistic view of herbal medicine.

- A fusion of wisdom on holistic healing using in-depth herb profiles: Learn how to create holistic treatments that address specific health conditions using the "Encyclopedia" in-depth herb descriptions. Integrate what you learn about the characteristics, applications, and energetic aspects of herbs into your health routines.

- A Complete Herbal Toolkit for Crafting Accurate Remedies: You may create a thorough herbal toolbox that equips you to handle a variety of health conditions by combining the lessons from all three books. Learn how to construct precise medicines by combining the concepts of herbal antibiotics, making preparations, and in-depth plant profiles.

11.3.2 A Bridge between Wisdom and Healing: Understanding Plant Energetics

The "Encyclopedia" explores the idea of plant energetics, a comprehensive method that takes into account how herbs affect the body's energetic equilibrium. You'll develop a better grasp of how herbs interact with the body on many levels by fusing this information with the knowledge from the previous books.

- Enhancing Holistic Wellness: Integration for Empowerment: You are developing a holistic approach to well-being by fusing the knowledge from the "Encyclopedia of Herbal Medicine" and other books. You're building a strong foundation for thorough recovery by using the knowledge of herbal antibiotics, making remedies, and thorough herb profiles.

- The Journey of Integration: Fostering Wisdom and Empowerment: You are starting a journey of integration that will take you to empowerment and wisdom by combining the information from these three books. With the help of this synthesis of knowledge, you can confidently explore the realm of herbal medicine and make decisions that are best for your health.

You will obtain a better grasp of the holistic therapeutic potential of herbs as a result of this investigation of the "Encyclopedia of Herbal Medicine." Join us as we continue to include information because we want to provide you with a thorough understanding of herbal medicine that supports your body and soul.

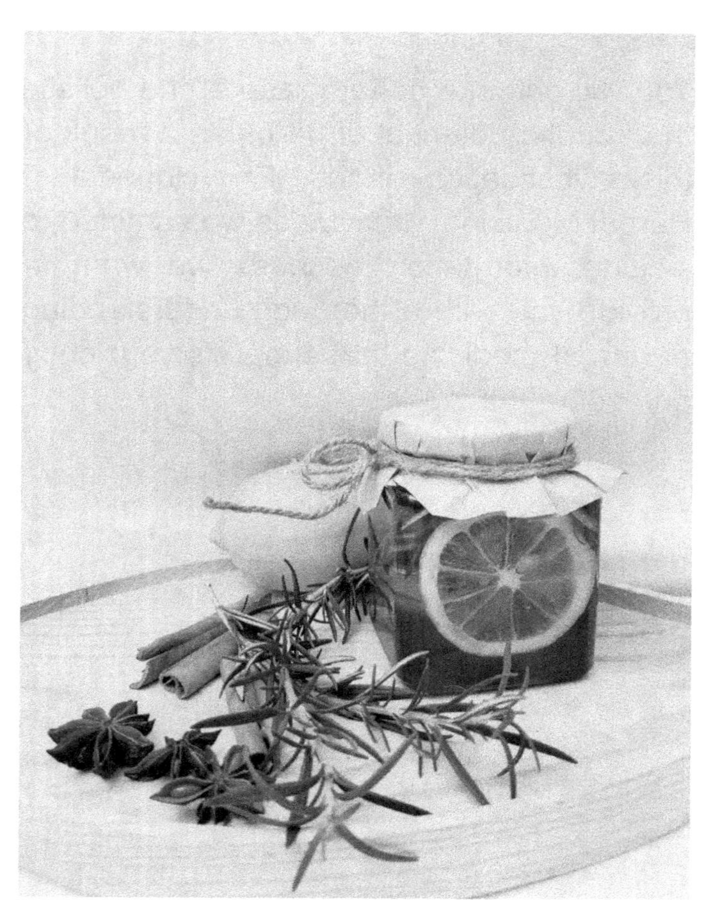

CHAPTER TWELVE: Your Herbal Journey: A Path to Wellness

12.1 Integrating Nature's Wisdom with Herbal Healing in Everyday Life

In this last chapter, we summarize the key points from the three volumes' treatment of herbal medicine as a whole. We'll look at ways to smoothly incorporate the knowledge you obtain from these sources into your day-to-day activities, promoting a holistic approach to well-being that respects both custom and contemporary knowledge.

12.1.1 The Path of Integration: A Comprehensive Approach to Healing

By fusing the knowledge of herbal antibiotics, creating remedies, in-depth herb profiles, and more, consider the integration trip you've walked. Recognize the role that each piece of knowledge plays in the bigger picture of holistic well-being.

- Daily Rituals and Practices for a Herbalist Lifestyle: Learn how to include herbal healing in your daily life. Learn how to include herbs in your daily rituals, from morning to nighttime routines, to foster a healthy relationship with nature.

- Herbs as Self-Care Allies: Nurturing the Mind, Body, and Spirit: Learn how herbs may help you take care of yourself by supporting your physical, emotional, and spiritual well-being. Learn how to utilize herbs for nourishing, calming, balancing emotions, and preserving healthy health.

- Developing Intuition: Paying Attention to Your Body's Wisdom: You'll acquire a stronger intuitive sense of knowing what your body requires as a result of the information you learn from these sources.

Discovering how to listen to the messages your body sends can help you choose herbs and treatments that work with your particular constitution.

- Building a Personal Herbal Pharmacy: Your Wellness Toolkit: Learn how to build a customized herbal apothecary packed with medications suited to your medical need. Learn how to choose, make, and store herbal remedies so you can better handle a variety of health issues.

- Sharing the Knowledge: Giving Others Access to Herbal Information: You have the chance to teach people about herbal wisdom as you apply it to your daily life. Learn how to use herbal insights to empower friends, family, and communities, promoting well-being and a feeling of connection.

12.1.2 The continuation of your herbal journey: continuous improvement:

Your herbal journey continues; it is a continuous process of education, development, and investigation. Accept the dynamic character of herbal medicine and keep developing your relationship with nature.

You'll learn how to accept herbal medicine as a holistic route to well-being that jives with your beliefs and goals via this last chapter. Join us as we complete this integrative journey, driven by the goal to provide you with the skills, information, and motivation to promote your well-being using the knowledge of nature's cures.

12.2 Making a Custom Herbal Protocol for Optimal Well-Being

We go into the process of developing a customized herbal regimen catered to your particular well-being in this portion of the last chapter. You'll acquire the skills necessary to create a wellness plan that aids in your pursuit of holistic health by combining the three books' ideas into one coherent strategy.

12.2.1 The Power of Personalization: Respecting Your Uniqueness

Understand the significance of establishing a tailored herbal regimen that respects your unique constitution, health objectives, and preferences. Recognize that achieving health is a very individual process, and your treatment should reflect that.

- Identifying Your Needs for Wellness: Mind, Body, and Spirit: Investigate the process of determining your physical, emotional, and spiritual well-being requirements. Recognize the areas in which herbal assistance might help you feel more balanced and vibrant overall.

- Integrating Herbal Antibiotic Wisdom: Boosting Immune Health: Incorporate the lessons learned from "Herbal Antibiotics" into your approach. Learn how to integrate antimicrobial herbs to strengthen your immune system's resistance to bacterial threats.

- Making Personalized Herbal Preparations: Promoting Self-Care: Explore the process of creating personalized herbal remedies that address your unique health issues, building on the information provided in "The Modern Herbal Dispensatory." Learn how to use your selected herbs to make teas, tinctures, salves, and other things.

12.2.2 Using Comprehensive Herb Profiles to Address Root Causes

Use the comprehensive herb profiles in the "Encyclopedia of Herbal Medicine" to tackle the underlying causes of your health issues. Learn about the energetics of herbs and how they affect the particular constitution of your body.

- Adopting Daily Rituals as Part of a Holistic Lifestyle Approach: Learn how to incorporate wellness-promoting daily routines into your lifestyle to complement herbal treatment. Promote a holistic approach to health by including herbs in your diet, self-care routines, and moments of mindfulness.

- Taking Action Through Self-Knowledge: Paying Attention to Your Body's Wisdom: You'll develop a closer connection with your body's knowledge as you establish and adhere to your herbal prescription. Discover how to decipher its messages, then modify your protocol as your requirements change.

- Continuous Development and Evolution: A Lifetime Journey: Your herbal regimen is a dynamic guide that changes as you do. Recognize that achieving well-being is a dynamic process and that your routine may need to change as your needs and goals change.

You'll obtain a comprehensive grasp of how to incorporate herbal knowledge into your everyday life via this investigation of developing a customized herbal program. Join us as we help you create a special route to wellness that embraces the efficacy of natural cures and gives you the ability to flourish on all levels of your existence.

12.3 Long-Term Health and Vitality: A Holistic Approach

This chapter's last section explores the idea of taking a comprehensive approach to long-term health and vitality. You'll have the means to nurture long-lasting well-being and energy by fusing the lessons from the three books and adopting a thorough wellness philosophy.

12.3.1 Taking care of one's mind, body, and spirit in a holistic manner

Recognize the fundamentals of holistic health, which include your mental, physical, and spiritual well-being. Investigate the connections between the contributions made by each aspect of your existence to your total vitality.

- Wellness Beyond Symptom Relief: The Continuum of Care: Instead of focusing on treating symptoms, adopt a continuum-based approach to health cultivation. Learn to prioritize self-care, balance, and preventative actions above only dealing with immediate health issues.

- Including Herbal Knowledge in Daily Life: A Wellness Lifestyle: Learn how to implement herbal knowledge into your everyday life. Accept herbs as companions in preserving vitality, from immune system support to stress management, from nourishing digestion to encouraging emotional well-being.

- Herbal Nutrition and Mindful Eating: Fueling Your Vitality: Examine how mindful eating may promote vitality. Learn how to add healthy herbs to your food to provide you with not only bodily but also energy and emotional nutrition.

- Getting in Touch with Vitality Through Movement and Nature: Recognize the value of activity and time spent in nature for fostering vitality. Learn how being in nature, using herbal treatments, and moving mindfully may improve your connection to life force energy.

- Balancing Rest, Restoration, and Action: Holistic Self-Care: Learn the skill of comprehensive self-care, which entails striking a balance between active participation and restorative activities. Know how your total vitality is affected by herbal medicines, meditation, sleep, and enjoyable hobbies.

- Developing Resilience: Accepting Change in Life with Grace: Accept the idea that resilience is a crucial aspect of long-term health. Learn to manage obstacles and transitions with grace, using the knowledge of herbs and holistic methods.

- A Lifelong Vitality Journey: The Integration of Wisdom: You're starting a lifetime adventure when you embrace a holistic approach to long-term health and vitality. You are given the ability to travel on this trip with knowledge, awareness, and a strong connection to nature's cures by combining the lessons from the three books.

You will learn the skills necessary to promote a life filled with vigor, happiness, and connections via this investigation of a holistic approach to long-term health and vitality. Come along as we wrap up our investigation to provide you with the information and skills you need to succeed on your herbal path to long-lasting vitality.

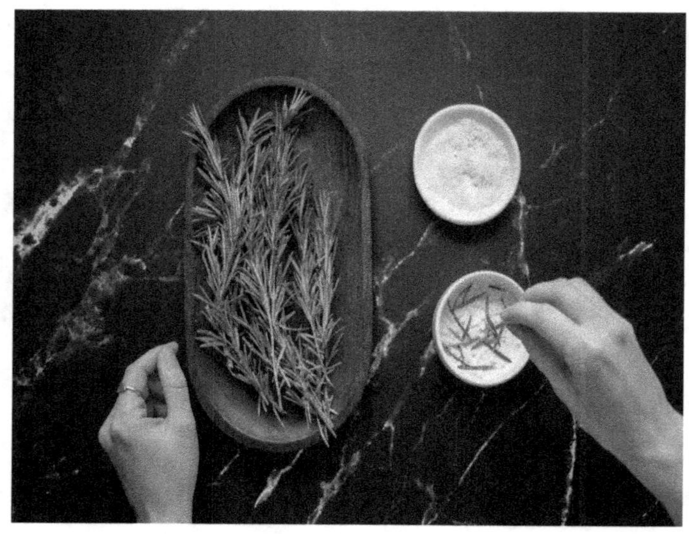

CONCLUSION

Promoting Wellness With Nature's Blessings

As we approach our destination, we take a moment to consider the tremendous knowledge and insights we have learned from "The Modern Herbal Dispensatory," "Herbal Antibiotics," and "Encyclopedia of Herbal Medicine." By combining these sources, we've started a comprehensive investigation into herbal medicine—a voyage that has outlined how to cultivate well-being using nature's many cures.

A Holistic Path to Healing: Harmonizing Tradition and Modern Understanding
Traditional herbal knowledge and cutting-edge scientific understanding have been combined to create a holistic approach to healing that respects the interdependence of all life. You've started a path that gives you the ability to control your health by adopting herbal antibiotics,

creating preparations, studying in-depth herb profiles, and more.

- The wisdom of nature as a source of empowerment: You've learned through this trip that the abundance of nature has a plethora of treatments that may boost your health and energy. You are now better able to connect with the medicinal properties of plants and develop a closer connection with nature thanks to the insights from these books.

- A Complete Wellness Toolkit: Personalized and Holistic Approaches: You now have a complete toolset for well-being, one that enables you to create treatments specific to your requirements, deal with both urgent and persistent issues and promote a holistic equilibrium of the mind, body, and spirit.

The continuation of wisdom from "A Lifelong Exploration Journey"

As you go, keep in mind that this trip is an ongoing exploration rather than a destination. As you include herbs into your everyday life, make educated decisions, and adopt a holistic approach to well-being, your knowledge will continue to grow and improve.

- Nature's Blessings: Promoting Wellness: A Lasting Legacy: These books' knowledge will live on forever, connecting you to a long line of herbalists, healers, and searchers who have used nature's abundance for health. You are preserving the tradition of holistic health and sustainable living by accepting this knowledge.

May you find motivation, strength, and comfort in the embrace of nature's cures as you go on your herbal adventure. You are well-equipped to foster well-being, energy, and a deep connection to nature with the skills, information, and insights you've learned. Accept this trip with an open mind, and may the abundance of nature's knowledge continue to enlighten and nourish you on the road to total well-being.

Key Takeaways from "Reflecting on the Holistic Journey"

As we reflect on the all-encompassing trip we've taken while reading "The Modern Herbal Dispensatory," "Herbal Antibiotics," and "Encyclopedia of Herbal Medicine," let's review the important takeaways that have widened your comprehension of herbal healing and wellbeing.

1. Integrating Traditional and Modern Values:
You now know how to combine conventional herbal knowledge with cutting-edge scientific knowledge. You've developed a balanced approach to herbal medicine that speaks to both traditional practices and modern demands by fusing information from various sources.

2. Natural antibiotics and immune boosters

You were first exposed to the idea of employing herbs as natural antibiotics in "Herbal Antibiotics." You've looked at plants with strong antibacterial characteristics and learned how they may help with bacterial problems and boost immunological health.

3. Making precise herbal preparations:

You gained knowledge of the art and science of creating herbal remedies from "The Modern Herbal Dispensatory". You now have newfound knowledge about choosing high-quality herbs, making extracts, teas, and tinctures, and developing personalized treatments for a variety of health issues.

4. Detailed Herb Profiles

Your knowledge was broadened by the "Encyclopedia of Herbal Medicine" since it included in-depth profiles of more than 550 herbs. Your comprehension of the traits, qualities, and applications of each plant has increased, enabling you to customize treatments to suit specific requirements.

5. Holistic Connection and Healing

You have adopted a holistic therapeutic approach throughout this trip, one that takes into account the interdependence of the mind, body, and spirit. You've discovered how to take care of your well-being via thoughtful activities, wholesome meals, exercise, and a strong connection to nature.

6. Self-Care Promotes Empowerment

You've learned that herbal medicine is a path toward self-care and empowerment as well as a focus on remedies. You've taken control of your health by developing a personal herbal pharmacy, including herbs in daily rituals, and paying attention to your body's wisdom.

7. Sustainable living and moral conduct

The value of ethical herbal practices and ecological living has also been stressed throughout this voyage. You have gained knowledge about ethical wildcrafting, environmentally beneficial methods, and how your decisions affect the environment and future generations.

8. Lifelong learning and evolution are topics Your journey continues; it is a continuous process of education, development, and discovery. You are creating a legacy of well-being that goes beyond yourself by continuing to develop your relationship with herbal knowledge.

May you take these important realizations ahead as you think about them with a feeling of empowerment and a renewed connection to nature's riches. You may promote a holistic approach to well-being—one that supports not just your physical health but also your mind, heart, and spirit—by accepting the advice presented in these books. With the information and experience you've learned, you'll continue on your road to holistic health as you travel toward optimal health and vitality.

Embracing Herbal Wisdom: Changing Lives and Health

After reading "The Modern Herbal Dispensatory," "Herbal Antibiotics," and "Encyclopedia of Herbal Medicine," we have reached the point where we can see the transformational potential of accepting herbal learning. The knowledge you learn from these sources has the power to alter not just your health but also the course of your whole life.

1. Knowledge Leads to Empowerment
You've discovered a wealth of information about the medicinal potential of plants by reading these books. With this information, you are better equipped to make choices about your health and move from being a passive receiver of treatment to an active participant in your road to wellness.

2. A Close Relationship with Nature
You've developed a stronger connection with nature thanks to herbal medicine. You've learned that the plants in your

immediate environment carry the secrets of sustaining and preserving your body, mind, and soul. This link with the Earth's plentiful offerings is spiritual and goes beyond simple physical cures.

3. Holistic health as a way of life
These books' knowledge has surpassed the limitations of medicine and transformed into a way of life that emphasizes holistic healing. You've developed a profoundly different perspective on self-care as a result of learning to see health as a synthesis of your physical, mental, emotional, and spiritual well-being.

4. An Individualized Wellness Plan:
You've developed a unique route to health by mixing knowledge from numerous sources. This route acknowledges that you are an original person with particular requirements. You've made the transition from depending only on outside answers to designing your health path.

5. Healing as a Process, Not a Goal:
You've learned from these books that mending is a process that never ends. Continuous learning, adaptability, and development are all parts of the process. With this viewpoint, you are freed from the need for instant treatments and can appreciate the progressive, transforming nature of herbal therapies.

6. Empowering Others: The Spread of Transformation:
Your transformation spreads when you apply herbal knowledge to your daily life. You encourage people to start their recovery journeys by imparting your wisdom and experiences. These individual changes may have a cumulative effect that creates a world that is healthier and more peaceful.

7. A Legacy of Wisdom and Good Health:
You are creating a legacy of well-being for yourself and future generations by embracing herbal knowledge. Your decisions, deeds, and experiences are woven into a story that honors the capacity

for natural healing and the intrinsic wisdom of the human spirit.

8. A Never-Ending Discovery Journey
This chapter is only the start of a never-ending voyage of discovery, not its conclusion. As you go through the complex terrain of health, energy, and development, the knowledge of herbs will continue to reveal itself, change, and astound you.

Adopting herbal knowledge results in a transformation that extends beyond improvements in physical health; it penetrates the soul, enlivens the spirit, and changes how you see life in general. May the healing power of herbs lead you into a life of vitality, well-being, and close connection to the environment as you continue to embrace this transforming path.

Appendix

Resources and References

Further Reading: Recommended Books, Journals, and Online Resources

As you continue your exploration of herbal healing and wellness, here are some recommended resources to further enrich your knowledge:

Books

- "The Herbal Medicine-Maker's Handbook: A Home Manual" by James Green
- "Rosemary Gladstar's Medicinal Herbs: A Beginner's Guide" by Rosemary Gladstar

- "The Herbal Apothecary: 100 Medicinal Herbs and How to Use Them" by JJ Pursell
- "Alchemy of Herbs: Transform Everyday Ingredients into Foods and Remedies That Heal" by Rosalee de la Forêt

Journals

- "HerbalGram" by the American Botanical Council
- "Journal of Ethnopharmacology"
- "Phytomedicine"

Online Resources

- American Herbalists Guild (AHG): www.americanherbalistsguild.com
- United Plant Savers: www.unitedplantsavers.org
- Herbal Academy: www.herbalacademy.com

Scientific References and Studies Supporting Herbal Medicine

Here are a few key scientific references and studies that provide evidence of the efficacy of herbal medicine:

1. Williamson EM. (2003). Synergy and other interactions in phytomedicines. Phytomedicine, 10(5), 401-403.
2. Gertsch, J., & Viveros-Paredes, J. M. (2010). The endocannabinoid system and plant-derived cannabinoids in diabetes and diabetic complications. British Journal of Pharmacology, 160(3), 511-523.
3. Yang, F., Li, S., Hu, M., & Wang, Y. (2020). Antiviral activity of baicalin against influenza A (H1N1/H3N2) virus in cell culture and mice and its inhibition of neuraminidase. Archives of Virology, 165(4), 801-811.
4. Thosar, N., Basak, S., & Bahadur, S. (2021). Traditional Indian herbs and their potential antiviral activity: A systematic

review. Journal of Traditional and Complementary Medicine, 11(4), 273-284.

Please note that the field of herbal medicine is constantly evolving, and new research is continuously being conducted. Consult reputable journals, publications, and institutions for the latest scientific insights into herbal remedies.

By exploring these additional resources and referencing scientific studies, you'll be able to deepen your understanding of herbal medicine and continue to make informed choices on your wellness journey.